Ben Stacy Jerrik (Ed.)

Parents' Rights Movement

Ben Stacy Jerrik (Ed.)

Parents' Rights Movement

Children, Lesbians, COLAGE, chapter, lesbian

Part Press

Contents

Articles

References

Parents'_rights_movement

The **Parents' rights movement** is a civil rights movement whose members are primarily interested in issues affecting fathers, mothers and children related to family law, including child custody.

Parents' rights advocates claim that many parents' parental rights are unnecessarily terminated, and that children are separated from fathers and mothers and adopted through the actions of family courts and government social service agencies seeking to meet their own targets, rather than looking at the merits of each case.[1] Parental rights activists state that employees of the Massachusetts Department of Social Services (DSS) take children away from their parents without cause.[2] They add that these employees, who they assert have improperly received immunity from the Massachusetts Supreme Court,[3] threaten mothers with the loss of their children to coerce them into divorcing their husbands[4] and attending support groups.[5] They state that these support groups serve the dual purpose of allowing the associates of the DSS employees to receive additional government funding for running the support groups, and allowing the DSS employees to gain information used to take children away from their parents.[5] Parental rights advocates state that abuse of power has occurred[2] and that vested interest has played a role.[5]

In June 2007, UK parents' rights advocates criticized the local court, claiming that it was treating children as adoptable commodities, that decisions were made on lack of evidence and perjury, and that courtroom secrecy was harming families and children.[6]

References

[1] "Unwarranted Adoptions" (http://news.bbc.co.uk/1/hi/help/3662494.stm). BBC. 2004-09-28. . Retrieved 2007-06-05.

[2] Hession, Gregory (2003-01-06). "DSS Dirty Tricks Series" (http://www.massoutrage.com/dssdirtytricks.htm). MassOutrage.Com. . Retrieved 2007-04-27.

[3] Baskerville, Stephen (2004-06-06). "MASSACHUSETTS' FAMILY 'JUSTICE'" (http://www.newswithviews.com/Baskerville/stephen1. htm). NewsWithViews.com. . Retrieved 2007-05-07.

[4] Baskerville, Stephen (Summer 2003). "Divorce as Revolution" (http://www.fatherhoodcoalition.org/cpf/newreadings/2003/ Divorce_as_Revolution_SBsum03.htm). The Fatherhood Coalition, also Salisbury Review vol. 21 no. 4. . Retrieved 2007-03-22.

[5] Moore, Nev (2003-07-29). "Inside A 'Batterers Program' for 'Abused' Women" (http://www.fatherhoodcoalition.org/cpf/newreadings/ 2003/NevIndepHouse0307.htm). The Fatherhood Coalition. . Retrieved 2007-04-17.

[6] "Parents' Rights Advocates Criticize Local Court" (http://news.bbc.co.uk/media/avdb/regions/west_yorkshire/video/98000/nb/ 98414_16x9_nb.ram). BBC. . Retrieved 2007-06-06.

Civil_rights_movement

The **civil rights movement** was a worldwide political movement for equality before the law occurring between approximately 1950 and 1980. In many situations it took the form of campaigns of civil resistance aimed at achieving change by nonviolent forms of resistance. In some situations it was accompanied, or followed, by civil unrest and armed rebellion. The process was long and tenuous in many countries, and many of these movements did not fully achieve their goals although, the efforts of these movements did lead to improvements in the legal rights of previously oppressed groups of people.

Civil rights movement in Northern Ireland

Further information: Northern Ireland Civil Rights Association

Northern Ireland is a province of the United Kingdom which has witnessed violence over many decades, mainly because of sectarian tensions between the Catholic and Protestant community, known as the Troubles.

The civil rights struggle in Northern Ireland can be traced to Catholics in Dungannon who were fighting for equal access to public housing for the members of the Catholic community, led by Austin Currie. This domestic issue would not have led to a fight for civil rights were it not for the fact that being a registered householder was a qualification for local government franchise in Northern Ireland. This substantial contribution made by women is often erased from the general history of Northern Ireland, primarily because the country still has a Protestant majority and a conservative culture where people often overlook the role of women in the political sphere.[1]

On a broader and more organized front, in January 1964, the Campaign for Social Justice (CSJ) was officially launched in Belfast.[2] This organization took over women's struggle for better housing and committed itself to ending discrimination in employment. The CSJ promised the Catholic community that their cries would be heard. They challenged the government and promised that they would take their case to the Commission for Human Rights in Strasbourg and to the United Nations.[3]

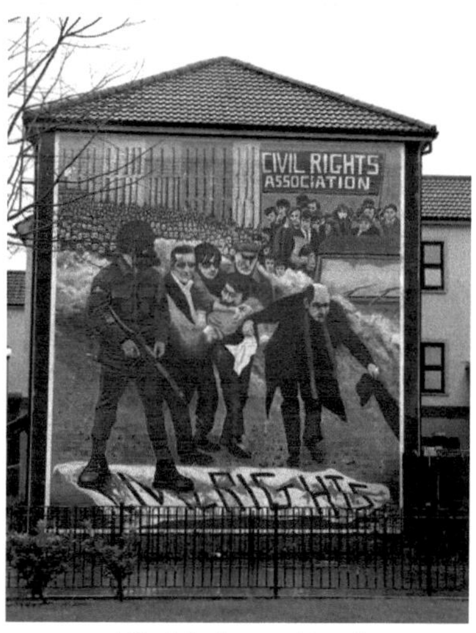

A Bloody Sunday memorial mural

Having started with basic domestic issues, the civil rights struggle in Northern Ireland escalated to a full scale movement that found its embodiment in the Northern Ireland Civil Rights Association. The NICRA campaigned in the late sixties and early seventies, consciously modelling itself on the American civil rights movement and using similar methods of civil resistance. Empowered by what African Americans were doing, the movement organized marches and protests to demand better conditions for the minority of Catholics who lived in the Protestant state.

NICRA originally had five main demands:

- one man, one vote
- an end to discrimination in housing
- an end to discrimination in local government
- an end to the gerrymandering of district boundaries, which limited the effect of Catholic voting

- the disbandment of the B-Specials, an entirely Protestant Police reserve, perceived as sectarian.

All of these specific demands were aimed at an ultimate goal that had been the one of women at the very beginning: the end of discrimination.

Civil rights activists all over Northern Ireland soon launched a campaign of civil resistance. There was opposition from Loyalists, who were aided by the Royal Ulster Constabulary (RUC), Northern Ireland's Police Force. At this point, the RUC was over 90% Protestant. Violence escalated, resulting in the rise of the Provisional Irish Republican Army (IRA) from the Catholic community, a group reminiscent of those from the War of Independence and the Civil War that occurred in the 1920s that had launched a campaign of violence to end British rule in Northern Ireland. Loyalist paramilitaries countered this with a defensive campaign of violence and the British government responded with a policy of internment without trial of suspected IRA members. For more than three hundred people, the internment lasted several years. The huge majority of those interned by the British forces were Catholic. In 1978, in a case brought by the government of the Republic of Ireland against the government of the United Kingdom, the European Court of Human Rights ruled that the interrogation techniques approved for use by the British army on internees in 1971 amounted to "inhuman and degrading" treatment.

Although it is common knowledge that, for a time, the aims of the Republicans was for their military division, the IRA, and the NICRA to converge, the two bodies never did so. The IRA told the Republicans to join in the civil rights movement but it never controlled the NICRA. The Northern Ireland Civil Rights Association fought for the end of discrimination toward Catholics and was happy to do so within the British state.[4] Republican leader Gerry Adams explained subsequently that Catholics saw that it was possible for them to have their demands heard. He wrote that "we were able to see an example of the fact that you didn't just have to take it, you could fight back".[3] For an account and critique of the civil rights movement in Northern Ireland, reflecting on the ambiguous link between the causes of civil rights and opposition to the union with the United Kingdom, see the work of Richard English.[5]

One of the most important events in the era of civil rights in Northern Ireland took place in Derry, which escalated the conflict from peaceful civil disobedience to armed conflict. The Battle of the Bogside started on 12 August when an Apprentice Boys, a Protestant order, parade passed through Waterloo Place, where a large crowd was gathered at the mouth of William Street, on the edge of the Bogside. Different accounts describe the first outbreak of violence, with reports stating that it was either an attack by youth from the Bogside on the RUC, or fighting broke out between Protestants and Catholics. The violence escalated and barricades were erected. Proclaiming this district to be the Free Derry, Bogsiders carried on fights with the RUC for days using stones and petrol bombs. The government finally withdrew the RUC and replaced it with the army, which disbanded the crowds of Catholics who were barricaded in the Bogside.[6]

Bloody Sunday, 30 January 1972, in Derry is seen by some as a turning point in the civil rights movement. Up to that day, so one interpretation goes, Catholics were trying to peacefully resolve the problem, but they were ignored and fights broke out. Fourteen unarmed Catholic civil rights marchers protesting against internment were shot dead by the British army and many were left wounded on the streets.

The peace process has made significant gains in recent years. Through open dialogue from all parties, a state of ceasefire by all major paramilitary groups has lasted. A strong economy and more opportunities for all citizens has greatly improved Northern Ireland's standard of living. Civil rights issues have become far less of a concern for many in Northern Ireland over the past twenty years as laws and policies protecting their rights and forms of affirmative action have been implemented for all government offices and many private businesses. Tensions still exist in some corners of the province, but the vast majority of citizens are no longer affected by the violence that once paralyzed the province.

Independence movements in Africa

A wave of independence movements in Africa crested in the 1960s, which included the Angolan War of Independence, the Guinea-Bissauan Revolution, the war of liberation in Mozambique and the struggle against apartheid in South Africa. This wave of struggles re-energised pan-Africanism and led to the founding of the Organization of African Unity (OAU) in 1963.

Canada's Quiet Revolution

The 1960s brought intense political and social change to the Canadian province of Quebec, with the election of Liberal Premier Jean Lesage after the death of Maurice Duplessis, whose government was widely viewed as corrupt.[7] These changes included secularization of the education and health care systems, which were both heavily controlled by the Roman Catholic Church, whose support for Duplessis and his perceived corruption had angered many Québecois. Policies of the Liberal government also sought to give Quebec more economic autonomy, such as the nationalization of Hydro-Québec and the creation of public companies for the mining, forestry, iron/steel and petroleum industries of the province. Other changes included the creation of the *Régie des Rentes du Québec* (Quebec Pension Plan) and new labour codes that made unionizing easier and gave workers the right to strike.

The social and economic changes of the Quiet Revolution gave life to the Quebec sovereignty movement, as more and more Québecois saw themselves as a distinctly culturally different from the rest of Canada. The segregationist Parti Québecois was created in 1968 and won the 1976 Quebec general election. They enacted legislation meant to enshrine French as the language of business in the province, while also controversially restricting the usage of English on signs and restricting the eligibility of students to be taught in English.

A radical strand of French Canadian nationalism produced the Front de libération du Québec (FLQ), which since 1963 has been using terrorism to make Quebec a sovereign nation. In October 1970, in response to the arrest of some of its members earlier in the year, the FLQ kidnapped British diplomat James Cross and Quebec's Minister of Labour Pierre Laporte, whom they later killed. The then Canadian Prime Minister Pierre Elliott Trudeau, himself a French Canadian, invoked the War Measures Act, declared martial law in Quebec, and arrested the kidnappers by the end of the year.

Civil rights movement in the United States

The civil rights movement in the United States includes noted legislation and organized efforts to abolish public and private acts of racial discrimination African Americans and other disadvantaged groups between 1954 to 1968, particularly in the southern United States. It is sometimes referred to as the Second Reconstruction era, echoing the unresolved issues of the Reconstruction era in the United States (1863–1877).

Ethnicity equity issues

Integrationism

After 1890 the system of Jim Crow, disenfranchisement, and second class citizenship degraded the citizenship rights of African Americans, especially in the South. It was the nadir of American race relations. There were three main aspects: racial segregation – upheld by the United States Supreme Court decision in *Plessy v. Ferguson* in 1896 –, legally mandated by southern governments—voter suppression or disfranchisement in the southern states, and private acts of violence and mass racial violence aimed at African Americans, unhindered or encouraged by government authorities. Although racial discrimination was present nationwide, the combination of law, public and private acts of discrimination, marginal economic opportunity, and violence directed toward African Americans in the southern states became known as Jim Crow.

Noted strategies employed prior to 1955 included litigation and lobbying attempts by the National Association for the Advancement of Colored People (NAACP). These efforts were a hallmark of the American Civil Rights Movement from 1896 to 1954. However, by 1955, blacks became frustrated by gradual approaches to implement desegregation by federal and state governments and the "massive resistance" by whites. The black leadership adopted a combined strategy of direct action with nonviolent resistance known as civil disobedience. The acts of civil disobedience produced crisis situations between

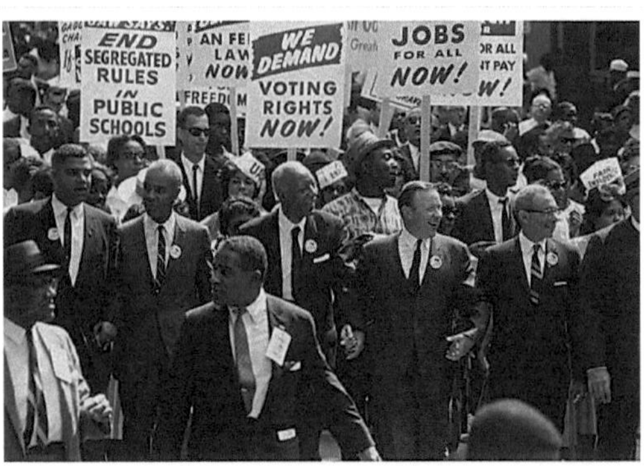

March on Washington for Jobs and Freedom

practitioners and government authorities. The authorities of federal, state, and local governments often had to act with an immediate response to end crisis situations – sometimes in the practitioners' favor. Some of the different forms of protests and/or civil disobedience employed included boycotts, as successfully practiced by the Montgomery Bus Boycott (1955–1956) in Alabama which gave the movement one of its more famous icons in Rosa Parks; "sit-ins", as demonstrated by the influential Greensboro sit-in (1960) in North Carolina; and marches, as exhibited by the Selma to Montgomery marches (1965) in Alabama. The evidence of changing attitudes could also be seen around the country, where small businesses sprang up supporting the civil rights movement, such as New Jersey's notable Everybody's Luncheonette.[8]

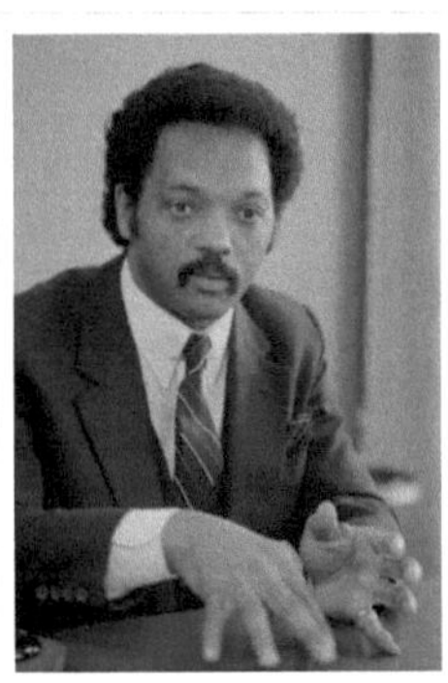

Jesse Jackson has fought for civil rights as his life's work.

The most illustrious march is probably the March on Washington for Jobs and Freedom. It is best remembered for the glorious speech Martin Luther King, Jr. gave, in which the "I have a dream" part turned into a national text and eclipsed the troubles the organizers had to bring to march forward. It had been a fairly complicated affair to bring together various leaders of civil rights, religious and labor groups. As the name of the march tells us, many compromises had to be made in order to unite the followers of so many different causes. The "March on Washington for Jobs and Freedom" emphasized the combined purposes of the march and the goals that each of the leaders aimed at. These leaders, informally named the Big Six, were A. Philip Randolph, Roy Wilkins, Martin Luther King Jr., Whitney Young, James Farmer and John Lewis. Although they came from different political horizons, these leaders were intent on the peacefulness of the march, which even had its own marshal to ensure that the event would be peaceful and respectful of the law.[9] The success of the march is still being debated but one aspect has been raised in the last few years: the misrepresentation of women. A lot of feminine civil rights groups had participated in the organization of the march but when it came to actual activity, women were denied the right to speak and were relegated to figurative roles in the back of the stage. As some female participants have noticed, the March can be remembered for the "I Have a Dream" speech but for most female activists it was a new awakening, forcing black women not only to fight for civil rights but also to engage in the Feminist movement.[10]

Noted achievements of the civil rights movement in this area include the judicial victory in the *Brown v. Board of Education* case that nullified the legal article of "separate but equal" and made segregation legally impermissible, passage of the Civil Rights Act of 1964[11] that banned discrimination in employment practices and public accommodations, passage of the Voting Rights Act of 1965 that restored voting rights, and passage of the Civil Rights Act of 1968 that banned discrimination in the sale or rental of housing.

Black Power

By 1965, the emergence of the Black Power movement (1966–1975) began to gradually eclipse the original "integrated power" aims of the civil rights movement that had been espoused by Martin Luther King, Jr.. Advocates of Black Power argued for black self-determination, and asserted that the assimilation inherent in integration robs Africans of their common heritage and dignity; e.g., the theorist and activist Omali Yeshitela argues that Africans have historically fought to protect their lands, cultures and freedoms from European colonialists, and that any integration into the society which has stolen another people and their wealth is actually an act of treason.

Today, most Black Power advocates have not changed their self-sufficiency argument. Racism still exists worldwide and it is believed by some that blacks in the United States, on the whole, did not assimilate into U.S. "mainstream" culture, either by King's integration measures or by the self-sufficiency measures of Black Power—rather, blacks arguably became even more oppressed, this time partially by "their own" people in a new black stratum of the middle class and the ruling class. Black Power's advocates generally argue that the reason for this stalemate and further oppression of the vast majority of U.S. blacks is because Black Power's objectives have not had the opportunity to be fully carried through.

One of the most public manifestations of the Black Power movement took place in the 1968 Olympics, when two African-Americans stood on the podium doing a Black Power salute. This act is still remembered today as the 1968 Olympics Black Power salute.

Chicano Movement

The Chicano Movement, also known as the Chicano Civil Rights Movement, Mexican-American Civil Rights Movement and *El Movimiento*, was the part of the American Civil Rights Movement that sought political empowerment and social inclusion for Mexican-Americans around a generally nationalist argument. The Chicano movement blossomed in the 1960s and was active through the late 1970s in various regions of the U.S. The movement had roots in the civil rights struggles that had preceded it, adding to it the cultural and generational politics of the era.

The early heroes of the movement—Rodolfo Gonzales in Denver, Colorado and Reies Tijerina in New Mexico—adopted a historical account of the preceding hundred and twenty-five years that had obscured much of Mexican-American history. Gonzales and Tijerina embraced a nationalism that identified the failure of the United States government to live up to its promises in the Treaty of Guadalupe Hidalgo. In that account, Mexican-Americans were a conquered people who simply needed to reclaim their birthright and cultural heritage as part of a new nation, which later became known as Aztlán.

That version of the past did not, but take into account the history of those Mexicans who had immigrated to the United States. It also gave little attention to the rights of undocumented immigrants in the United States in the 1960s— which is not surprising, since immigration did not have the political significance it later acquired. It was a decade later when activists, such as Bert Corona in California, embraced the rights of undocumented workers and helped broaden the movement to include their issues.

When the movement dealt with practical problems in the 1960s, most activists focused on the most immediate issues confronting Mexican-Americans; unequal educational and employment opportunities, political disfranchisement, and police brutality. In the heady days of the late 1960s, when the student movement was active around the globe, the Chicano movement brought about more or less spontaneous actions, such as the mass walkouts by high school students in Denver and East Los Angeles in 1968 and the Chicano Moratorium in Los Angeles in 1970.

The movement was particularly strong at the college level, where activists formed MEChA, *Movimiento Estudiantil Chicano de Aztlán*, which promoted Chicano Studies programs and a generalized ethno-nationalist agenda.

American Indian Movement

At a time when peaceful sit-ins were a common protest tactic, the American Indian Movement (AIM) takeovers in their early days were noticeably violent. Some appeared to be spontaneous outcomes of protest gatherings, but others included armed seizure of public facilities, such as in the Wounded Knee incident.

The Alcatraz Island occupation of 1969, although commonly associated with NAM, pre-dated the organization, but was a catalyst for its formation.

In 1970, AIM occupied abandoned property at the Naval Air Station near Minneapolis, Minnesota. In July 1971, it assisted in a takeover of the Winter Dam, Lac Courte Oreilles, and Wisconsin. When activists took over the Bureau of Indian Affairs Headquarters in Washington D.C. in November 1972, they sacked the building and 24 people were arrested. Activists occupied the Custer County Courthouse in 1973, though police routed the occupation after a riot took place.

In 1973 activists and military forces confronted each other in the Wounded Knee incident. The standoff lasted 71 days, and two men died in the violence.

Gender equity issues

If the period associated with first-wave feminism focused upon absolute rights such as suffrage (which led to women attaining the right to vote in the early part of the 20th century), the period of the second-wave feminism was concerned with the issues such as changing social attitudes and economic, reproductive, and educational equality (including the ability to have careers in addition to motherhood, or the right to choose not to have children) between the genders and addressed the rights of female minorities. The new feminist movement, which spanned from 1963 to 1982, explored economic equality, political power at all levels, professional equality, reproductive freedoms, sexuality, issues with the family, educational equality, sexuality, and many other issues.

LGBT rights and gay liberation

Since the mid-19th century in Germany, social reformers have used the language of civil rights to argue against the oppression of same-sex sexuality, same-sex emotional intimacy, and gender variance. Largely, but not exclusively, these LGBT movements have characterized gender variant and homosexually-oriented people as a minority group(s); this was the approach taken by the homophile movement of the 1940s, 50s and early 60s. With the rise of secularism in the West, an increasing sexual openness, women's liberation, the 1960s counterculture, and a range of new social movements, the homophile movement underwent a rapid growth and transformation, with a focus on building community and unapologetic activism which came to be known as the Gay Liberation.

The words "Gay Liberation" echoed "Women's Liberation"; the Gay Liberation Front consciously took its name from the "National Liberation Fronts" of Vietnam and Algeria, and the slogan "Gay Power", as a defiant answer to the rights-oriented homophile movement, was inspired by Black Power and Chicano Power. The GLF's statement of purpose explained:

> "We are a revolutionary group of men and women formed with the realization that complete sexual liberation for all people cannot come about unless existing social institutions are abolished. We reject society's attempt to impose sexual roles and definitions of our nature."

> — GLF statement of purpose

GLF activist Martha Shelley wrote,

> "We are women and men who, from the time of our earliest memories, have been in revolt against the sex-role structure and nuclear family structure."

> — "Gay is Good", Martha Shelley, 1970

Gay Liberationists aimed at transforming fundamental concepts and institutions of society, such as gender and the family. In order to achieve such liberation, consciousness raising and direct action were employed. Specifically, the word 'gay' was preferred to previous designations such as homosexual or homophile; some saw 'gay' as a rejection of the false dichotomy heterosexual/homosexual. Lesbians and gays were urged to "come out" and publicly reveal their sexuality to family, friends and colleagues as a form of activism, and to counter shame with gay pride. "Gay Lib" groups were formed in Australia, New Zealand, Germany, France, the UK, the US, Italy and elsewhere. The lesbian group Lavender Menace was also formed in the U.S. in response to both the male domination of other Gay Lib groups and the anti-lesbian sentiment in the Women's Movement. Lesbianism was advocated as a feminist choice for women, and the first currents of lesbian separatism began to emerge.

By the late 1970s, the radicalism of Gay Liberation was eclipsed by a return to a more formal movement that became known as the Gay and Lesbian Rights Movement.

German student movement

The civil rights movement in Germany was a left-wing backlash against the post-Nazi Party era of the country, which still contained many of the conservative policies of both that era and of the pre-World War I Kaiser monarchy. The movement mainly attracted disillusioned students and was largely a protest movement analogous to others around the globe during the late 1960s. It was largely a reaction against the perceived authoritarianism and hypocrisy of the German government and other Western governments and the poor living conditions of students. A wave of protests, some violent, swept Germany, further fueled by over-reaction by the police and encouraged by other near-simultaneous protest movements across the world. Following more than a century of conservatism among German students, the German student movement also marked a significant major shift to the left-wing and radicalization of student politics.

Ulrike Meinhof while still a journalist

France 1968

A general strike broke out across France in May 1968, which began to reach near-revolutionary proportions before being discouraged by the French Communist Party and finally suppressed by the government, which accused the communists of plotting against the Republic. Some philosophers and historians have argued that the rebellion was the single most important revolutionary event of the 20th century because it wasn't participated in by a lone demographic, such as workers or racial minorities, but was rather a purely popular uprising, superseding ethnic, cultural, age and class boundaries.

It began as a series of student strikes that broke out at a number of universities and high schools in Paris following confrontations with university administrators and the police. The de Gaulle administration's attempts to quash those strikes by further police action only inflamed the situation further, leading to street battles with the police in the Latin Quarter, followed by a general strike by students and ten million French workers, roughly two-thirds of the French workforce. The protests reached the point that de Gaulle created a military operations headquarters to deal with the unrest, dissolved the National Assembly and called for new parliamentary elections on 23 June 1968.

The government was close to collapse at that point and De Gaulle had even taken temporary refuge at an airforce base in Germany, but the revolutionary situation evaporated almost as quickly as it arose. Workers went back to their jobs, urged on by the Confédération Générale du Travail, the leftist union federation, and the Parti Communiste Français (PCF), the French Communist Party. When the elections were finally held in June, the Gaullist party emerged even stronger than before.

Most of the protesters espoused left-wing causes, communism or anarchism, and many saw the events as an opportunity to shake up the "old society" in many social aspects, including methods of education, sexual freedom and free love. A small minority of protesters, such as the Occident group, espoused far-right causes.

On 29 May, several hundred thousand protesters led by the CGT marched through Paris, chanting *"Adieu, de Gaulle!"*, "Goodby, de Gaulle!".

While the government appeared to be close to collapse, de Gaulle chose not to say *adieu*. Instead, after ensuring that he had sufficient loyal military units mobilized to back him if push came to shove, he went on the radio the following day (the national television service was on strike) to announce the dissolution of the National Assembly, with elections to follow on 23 June. He ordered workers to return to work, threatening to institute a state of emergency if they did not.

From that point, the revolutionary feeling of the students and workers faded away. Workers gradually returned to work or were ousted from their plants by the police. The national student union called off street demonstrations the government banned a number of left organizations, and the police retook the Sorbonne on 16 June. De Gaulle triumphed in the elections held in June and the crisis had ended.

Tlatelolco massacre, Mexico

The **Tlatelolco massacre**, also known as **Tlatelolco's Night** (from a book title), took place in the afternoon and night of October 2, 1968, in the Plaza de las Tres Culturas in the Tlatelolco section of Mexico City. The death toll remains uncertain, with some estimates placing the number of deaths in the thousands, but most reporting 200–300 deaths with many more wounded and several thousand arrested.

The massacre was preceded by months of political unrest in the Mexican capital, echoing student demonstrations and riots all over the world during 1968. Mexican students wanted to exploit the attention focused on Mexico City for the 1968 Summer Olympics. President Gustavo Díaz Ordaz, however, was determined to stop the demonstrations and, in September, ordered the army to occupy the campus of the National Autonomous University of Mexico, the largest university in Latin America. Students were beaten and arrested indiscriminately, causing Rector Javier Barros Sierra to resign in protest on September 23.

However, student demonstrators were not deterred and the demonstrations grew in size until October 2, when, after nine weeks of student strikes, 15,000 students from various universities marched through the streets of Mexico City carrying red carnations to protest the army's occupation of the university campus. By nightfall, 5,000 students and workers, many of them with spouses and children, had congregated outside an apartment complex in the Plaza de las Tres Culturas in Tlatelolco for what was supposed to be a peaceful rally. Among their chants were *México – Libertad – México – Libertad* ("Mexico – Liberty – Mexico –Liberty"). Rally organizers attempted to call off the protest when they noticed an increased military presence in the area.

The massacre began at sunset when army and police forces — equipped with armored cars and tanks — surrounded the square and began firing live rounds into the crowd, hitting not only the protesters, but also other bystanders uninvolved with the protest. Demonstrators and passersby alike, including children, were caught in the fire; soon, mounds of bodies lay on the ground. The killing continued through the night, with soldiers carrying out mopping-up operations on a house-to-house basis in the apartment buildings adjacent to the square. Witnesses to the event claim that the bodies were later removed in garbage trucks.

The official government explanation of the incident was that armed provocateurs among the demonstrators, stationed in buildings overlooking the crowd, had begun the firefight, causing security forces to return fire in self-defense.

Prague Spring

Prague Spring (Czech: *Pražské jaro*, Slovak: *Pražská jar*, Russian: пражская весна) was a period of political liberalization in Czechoslovakia starting on January 5, 1968, and running until August 20 of that year, when the Soviet Union and its Warsaw Pact allies (except for Romania) invaded the country.

During World War II, Czechoslovakia fell into the Soviet sphere of influence, the Eastern Bloc. Since 1948 there were no parties other than the Communist Party in the country and it was indirectly managed by the Soviet Union. Unlike other countries of Central and Eastern Europe, the communist take-over in Czechoslovakia in 1948 was, although as brutal as elsewhere, a genuine popular movement. Reform in the country did not lead to the convulsions seen in Hungary.

Towards the end of World War II Joseph Stalin wanted Czechoslovakia, and signed an agreement with Winston Churchill and Franklin D. Roosevelt that Prague would be liberated by the Red Army, despite the fact that the United States Army under General

21. AUGUSTA 1968
BOLI ZABITÍ ZBRAŇAMI
OKUPAČNÝCH ARMÁD

MICHAL HAMRÁK
JÁN HATALA
JOZEF KOLESÁR
JÁN LÁSZLÓ
LADISLAV MARTONÍK
IVAN SCHMIEDT

Prague Spring memorial plate in Košice, Slovakia

George S. Patton could have liberated the city earlier. This was important for the spread of pro-Russian (and pro-communist) propaganda that came right after the war. People still remembered what they felt as Czechoslovakia's betrayal by the West at the Munich Agreement. For these reasons, the people voted for communists in the 1948 elections, the last democratic poll to take place there for a long time.

From the middle of the 1960s, Czechs and Slovaks showed increasing signs of rejection of the existing regime. This change was reflected by reformist elements within the communist party by installing Alexander Dubček as party leader. Dubček's reforms of the political process inside Czechoslovakia, which he referred to as *Socialism with a human face*, did not represent a complete overthrow of the old regime, as was the case in Hungary in 1956. Dubček's changes had broad support from the society, including the working class, but was seen by the Soviet leadership as a threat to their hegemony over other states of the Eastern Bloc and to the very safety of the Soviet Union. Czechoslovakia was in the middle of the defensive line of the Warsaw Pact and its possible defection to the enemy was unacceptable during the Cold War.

However, a sizeable minority in the ruling party, especially at higher leadership levels, was opposed to any lessening of the party's grip on society and actively plotted with the leadership of the Soviet Union to overthrow the reformers. This group watched in horror as calls for multi-party elections and other reforms began echoing throughout the country.

Between the nights of August 20 and August 21, 1968, Eastern Bloc armies from five Warsaw Pact countries invaded Czechoslovakia. During the invasion, Soviet tanks ranging in numbers from 5,000 to 7,000 occupied the streets. They were followed by a large number of Warsaw Pact troops ranging from 200,000 to 600,000.

The Soviets insisted that they had been invited to invade the country, stating that loyal Czechoslovak Communists had told them that they were in need of "fraternal assistance against the counter-revolution". A letter which was found in 1989 proved an invitation to invade did indeed exist. During the attack of the Warsaw Pact armies, 72 Czechs and Slovaks were killed (19 of those in Slovakia) and hundreds were wounded (up to September 3, 1968). Alexander Dubček called upon his people not to resist. He was arrested and taken to Moscow, along with several of his colleagues.

1967 Australian Referendum

On 27 May 1967, Australians voted to amend their constitution, particularly removing Section 127, which had previously excluded Indigenous Australians from the census.

Notes

[1] Shannon, Catherine. "Women in Northern Ireland", in *Chattel, Servant or Citizen: Woman's Status in Church, State and Society*. Eds. Mary O'Dowd & Sabine Wichert. Historical Studies XIX (Belfast: Institute of Irish Studies Queen's University, 1995), 238–253.

[2] http://www.irelandseye.com/aarticles/history/events/conflict/bttc4.shtm

[3] Dooley, Brian. "Second Class citizens", in *Black and Green: The Fight for Civil Rights in Northern Ireland and Black America*. (London:Pluto Press, 1998), 28–48.

[4] Dooley, Brian. "Second Class citizens", in *Black and Green: The Fight for Civil Rights in Northern Ireland and Black America*. (London:Pluto Press, 1998), 28–48

[5] Richard English, "The Interplay of Non-violent and Violent Action in Northern Ireland, 1967-72", in Adam Roberts and Timothy Garton Ash (eds.), *Civil Resistance and Power Politics: The Experience of Non-violent Action from Gandhi to the Present*, Oxford University Press, 2009, ISBN 978-0-19-955201-6, pp. 75-90. (http://books.google.com/books?id=BxOQKrCe7UUC&dq=Civil+resistance+and+power+politics&source=gbs_navlinks_s)

[6] O'Dochartaigh, Niall. *From Civil Rights to Armalites: Derry and the Birth of the Irish Troubles* (Cork: Cork University Press, 1997), 1–18 and 111–152.

[7] http://www.wednesday-night.com/Duplessis.asp

[8] "Everybody's Luncheonette Camden, New Jersey" (http://www.freewebs.com/almasykusnyir/everybodys/index.htm). .

[9] Barber, Lucy. "In the Great Tradition: The March on Washington for Jobs ans Freedom, August 28, 1963," in *Marching on Washington: The Forging of an American Political Tradition*. (Berkeley: U of California Press, 2002), 141–178.

[10] Height,Dorothy. "We wanted the voice of a women to be heard": Black women and the 1963 March on Washington", in *Sisters in the Struggle: African American Women in the Civil Rights-Black Power Movement*. Eds. Collier. Thomas, Bettye and V.P. Franklin. (New York: NYU press, 2001), 83–91.

[11] Civil Rights Act of 1964 (http://finduslaw.com/ civil_rights_act_of_1964_cra_title_vii_equal_employment_opportunities_42_us_code_chapter_21)

Further reading

- Manfred Berg and Martin H. Geyer; *Two Cultures of Rights: The Quest for Inclusion and Participation in Modern America and Germany* Cambridge University Press, 2002
- Jack Donnelly and Rhoda E. Howard; *International Handbook of Human Rights* Greenwood Press, 1987
- David P. Forsythe; *Human Rights in the New Europe: Problems and Progress* University of Nebraska Press, 1994
- Joe Foweraker and Todd Landman; *Citizenship Rights and Social Movements: A Comparative and Statistical Analysis* Oxford University Press, 1997
- Mervyn Frost; *Constituting Human Rights: Global Civil Society and the Society of Democratic States* Routledge, 2002
- Marc Galanter; *Competing Equalities: Law and the Backward Classes in India* University of California Press, 1984
- Raymond D. Gastil and Leonard R. Sussman, eds.; *Freedom in the World: Political Rights and Civil Liberties, 1986-1987* Greenwood Press, 1987
- David Harris and Sarah Joseph; *The International Covenant on Civil and Political Rights and United Kingdom Law* Clarendon Press, 1995
- Steven Kasher; *The Civil Rights Movement: A Photographic History (1954–1968)* Abbeville Publishing Group (Abbeville Press, Inc.), 2000
- Francesca Klug, Keir Starmer, Stuart Weir; *The Three Pillars of Liberty: Political Rights and Freedoms in the United Kingdom* Routledge, 1996
- Fernando Santos-Granero and Frederica Barclay; *Tamed Frontiers: Economy, Society, and Civil Rights in Upper Amazonia* Westview Press, 2000

- Paul N. Smith; *Feminism and the Third Republic: Women's Political and Civil Rights in France, 1918-1940* Clarendon Press, 1996
- Jorge M. Valadez; *Deliberative Democracy: Political Legitimacy and Self-Determination in Multicultural Societies* Westview Press, 2000

External links

- We Shall Overcome: Historic Places of the Civil Rights Movement, a National Park Service *Discover Our Shared Heritage at* Travel Itinerary (http://www.nps.gov/nr/travel/civilrights/)
- A Columbia University Resource for Teaching African American History (http://www.amistadresource.org)
- Martin Luther King, Jr. and the Global Freedom Struggle, an encyclopedia presented by the Martin Luther King, Jr. Research and Education Institute at Stanford University (http://mlk-kpp01.stanford.edu/index.php/encyclopedia/encyclopedia_contents)
- Civil Rights (http://plato.stanford.edu/entries/civil-rights) entry by Andrew Altman in the *Stanford Encyclopedia of Philosophy*
- Martin Luther King, Jr. and the Global Freedom Struggle (http://mlk-kpp01.stanford.edu/index.php/encyclopedia/encyclopedia_contents/) ~ an online multimedia encyclopedia presented by the King Institute at Stanford University, includes information on over 1000 civil rights movement figures, events and organizations
- "CivilRightsTravel.com" (http://www.civilrightstravel.com) ~ a visitors guide to key sites from the civil rights movement
- The History Channel: Civil Rights Movement (http://www.history.com/topics/civil-rights-movement)
- Civil Rights: Beyond Black & White (http://www.life.com/image/first/in-gallery/22816/civil-rights-beyond-black--white) - slideshow by *Life magazine*
- Civil Rights in America: Connections to a Movement (http://civilrights.historybeat.com)

Child_custody

Child custody and **guardianship** are legal terms which are used to describe the legal and practical relationship between a parent and his or her child, such as the right of the parent to make decisions for the child, and the parent's duty to care for the child.

Following ratification of the United Nations Convention on the Rights of the Child in most countries, terms such as "residence" and "contact" (known as "visitation" in the United States) have superseded the concepts of "custody" and "access". Instead of a parent having "custody" of or "access" to a child, a child is now said to "reside" or have "contact" with a parent. For a discussion of the new international nomenclature, see parental responsibility.

Residence and contact issues typically arise in proceedings involving divorce (dissolution of marriage), annulment and other legal proceedings where children may be involved. In most jurisdictions the issue of which parent the child will reside with is determined in accordance with the best interests of the child standard.

Family law proceedings which involve issues of residence and contact often generate the most acrimonious disputes. While most parents cooperate when it comes to sharing their children and resort to mediation to settle a dispute, not all do. For those that engage in litigation, there seem to be few limits. Court filings quickly fill with mutual accusations by one parent against the other, including sexual, physical, and emotional abuse, brain-washing, parental alienation syndrome, sabotage, and manipulation. It is these infrequent yet difficult custody battles that become public via the media and sometimes distort the public's perceptions so that the issues appear more prevalent than they are and the court's response appear inadequate.

Forum shopping to gain advantage occurs both between nations and where laws and practices differ between areas within a nation, The Hague Convention seeks to avoid this, also in the United States of America, the Uniform Child Custody Jurisdiction and Enforcement Act was adopted by all 50 states, family law courts were forced to defer jurisdiction to the home state.

In some places, courts and legal professionals are beginning to use the term parenting schedule instead of custody and visitation. The new terminology eliminates the distinction between custodial and noncustodial parents, and also attempts to build upon the best interests of the children by crafting schedules that meet the developmental needs of the children. For example, younger children need shorter, more frequent time with parents, whereas older children and teenagers may demand less frequent shifts yet longer blocks of time with each parent.

Forms of custody

- Alternating custody is an arrangement whereby the child/children live for an extended period of time with one parent, and then for a similar amount of time with the other parent. While the child/children are with the parent, that parent retains sole authority over the child/children.
- Shared custody[1] is an arrangement whereby the child/children live for an extended period of time with one parent, and then for a similar amount of time with the other parent. Opposite to the Alternating custody both parents retains authority over the child/children.
- Bird's nest custody is an arrangement whereby the parents go back and forth from a residence in which the child/children reside, placing the burden of upheaval and movement on the parents rather than the child/children.
- Joint custody (*la garde conjointe* in French[2])is an arrangement whereby both parents have legal custody and/or both parents have physical custody.
- Sole custody (*la garde exclusive* in French[2]) is an arrangement whereby only one parent has physical and legal custody of a child.
- Split custody (*la garde divisée* in French[2]) is an arrangement whereby one parent has full time custody over some children, and the other parent has full custody over the other children.

- Third-party custody is an arrangement in whereby the children do not remain with either biological parent, and are placed under the custody of a third person.

Physical custody

Physical custody involves the day-to-day care of a child and establishes where a child will live. A parent with physical custody has the right to have his/her child live with him/her.

If a child lives with both parents, each parent shares **"joint physical custody"** and each parent is said to be a **"custodial parent"**. Thus, in joint physical custody, neither parent is said to be a "non-custodial parent."[3] In joint physical custody, actual lodging and care of the child is shared according to a court-ordered custody schedule (also known as a **"parenting plan"** or **"parenting schedule"**). In many cases, the term "visitation" is no longer used in this context, but rather is reserved to sole custody orders. Terms of art such as "primary custodial parent" and "primary residence" have no legal meaning other than for determining tax status, and both parents are still said to be "custodial parents".[4]

In some states, "joint physical custody" creates a presumption of "equal shared parenting". However, in most states, joint physical custody only creates an obligation to provide each of the parents with "significant periods" of physical custody so as to assure the child of "frequent and continuing contact" with both parents.[3] Courts have not clearly defined what "significant periods" and "frequent and continuous contact" mean, which requires parents to litigate to find out.

If a child lives with one parent, that parent has **"sole physical custody"** and is said to be the **"custodial parent"** whereas the other parent is said to be the **"non-custodial parent"**, but may have visitation rights or **"visitation"** with his/her child.[5]

Joint physical custody

Joint physical custody is a court order whereby custody of a child is awarded to both parties. In joint custody, both parents are *custodial parents* and neither parent is a non-custodial parents; in other words, the child has two custodial parents.

Many states recognize two forms of joint custody: joint physical custody, and joint legal custody. In joint legal custody, both parents share the ability to have access to educational, health, and other records, and have equal decision-making status where the welfare of the child is concerned.

In joint physical custody, which would include joint physical care, actual lodging and care of the child is shared according to a court-ordered custody schedule (also known as a *parenting plan* or *parenting schedule*). In many cases, the term *visitation* is no longer used in these circumstances, but rather is reserved to sole custody orders.[6] In some states joint physical custody creates a presumption of equal shared parenting, however in most states, joint physical custody creates an obligation to provide each of the parents with "significant periods" of physical custody so as to assure the child of "frequent and continuing contact" with both parents.[5] For example, states such as Alabama, California, and Texas do not necessarily require joint custody orders to result in substantially equal parenting time, whereas states such as Arizona, Georgia, and Louisiana do require joint custody orders to result in substantially equal parenting time where feasible.[7] Courts have not clearly defined what "significant periods" and "frequent and continuous contact" mean, which requires parents to litigate to find out.

It is important to note that joint physical custody and joint legal custody are different aspects of custody, and determination is often made separately in many states' divorce courts. E.g., it is possible to have joint legal custody, but for one parent to have sole physical custody In some states this is referred to as Custodial Parent and Non-Custodial Parent.

Also, where there is joint physical custody, terms of art such as "primary custodial parent" and "primary residence" have no legal meaning other than for determining tax status, and both parents are still custodial parents.[4]

Sole physical custody

Sole physical custody means that a child shall reside with and be under the supervision of one parent, subject to the power of the court to order visitation. Physical custody involves the day-to-day care of a child and establishes where a child will live. A parent with physical custody has the right to have his/her child live with him/her. If a child lives with only one parent, that parent has *sole physical custody* and is said to be the *custodial parent*. The other parent is said to be the *non-custodial parent*, and may have visitation rights or *visitation* with his/her child. [8] [5] [9] [10] [11]

Custodial parents

A *custodial parent* is a parent who is given physical and/or legal custody of a child by court order.

A *child-custody determination* means a judgment, decree, or other order of a court providing for the legal custody, physical custody, or visitation with respect to a child. The term includes a permanent, temporary, initial, and modification order. The term does not include an order relating to child support or other monetary obligation of an individual. [12] Where the child will live with both parents, joint physical custody is ordered , and both parent are custodial parents. Where the child will only live with one of the parents, sole physical custody is ordered , and the parent with which the child lives is the custodial parent, the other parent is the non-custodial parent.

Non-custodial parents

A *non-custodial parent* is a parent who does not have physical and/or legal custody of his/her child by court order.

A *child-custody determination* means a judgment, decree, or other order of a court providing for the legal custody, physical custody, or visitation with respect to a child. The term includes a permanent, temporary, initial, and modification order. The term does not include an order relating to child support or other monetary obligation of an individual. [12] Where the child will only live with one of the parents, sole physical custody is ordered, and the parent with which the child lives is the custodial parent, the other parent is the noncustodial parent. Note, however, where the child will live with both parents, joint physical custody is ordered , and both parent are custodial parents.

Criticism of policies concerning determination of child custody

Current policies concerning the determination of child custody have been criticized by certain groups. For more information and rationale, see the main article.

Before the 1970's child custody battles were almost unheard of in the United States. [13]

See also

- Coparenting
- Custodial parent
- Divorce
- Family court
- Family law
- Fathers' rights
- Legal custody
- Mothers' rights
- Noncustodial parent
- Parens patriae
- Parental alienation
- Parental alienation syndrome
- Parenting coordinator
- Parenting plan

- Physical custody
- Shared parenting
- Supervised visitation
- Tender years doctrine
- Ward of the state

By country or culture

- Child support by country
- Divorce in Judaism

United States

- Child custody laws in the United States

United Kingdom

- Residence in English law
- Shared residency in English law

References

[1] See *The Determination of Child Custody in the USA* (http://www.stanford.edu/group/psylawseminar/Child Custody in the USA (Page 1 of 5).htm) written by Joan B. Kelly, Ph.D. for Stanford University

[2] See the document published by the Canadian government here (http://www.justice.gov.nt.ca/pdf/Family/Custody_Access_FR.pdf). The document is also available for download here (https://docs.google.com/open?id=0B-iOqOKLc35PUFZJQi02Yy1TMkdzaDlOTXlmNDRCQQ)

[3] http://www.leginfo.ca.gov/cgi-bin/displaycode?section=fam&group=02001-03000&file=3000-3007)

[4] See e.g., In re Marriage of Rose and Richardson (App. 2 Dist. 2002) 126 Cal.App.4th 941. Moreover, several courts have also stated, "The term `primary physical custody' has no legal meaning." (In re Marriage of Biallas (1998) 65 Cal.App.4th 755, 759 citing Brody, Whealon, and Ruisi; see also In re Marriage of Richardson, 102 Cal.App.4th 941, 945, fn. 2; In re Marriage of Lasich (2002) 99 Cal.App.4th 702, 714

[5] "CA Codes (fam:3000-3007)" (http://www.leginfo.ca.gov/cgi-bin/displaycode?section=fam&group=02001-03000&file=3000-3007). Leginfo.ca.gov. . Retrieved 2012-01-09.

[6] "Custody | Divorce In California" (http://divorcelawca.com/category/custody/). Divorcelawca.com. . Retrieved 2012-01-09.

[7] Minnesota Presumptive Joint Physical Custody Group Report under House File 1262 (2008) Appendix B "State Definitions of Joint Physical Custody"

[8] "Section 30-3-151" (http://www.legislature.state.al.us/CodeofAlabama/1975/30-3-151.htm). Legislature.state.al.us. . Retrieved 2012-01-09.

[9] "Laws of New York" (http://public.leginfo.state.ny.us/menugetf.cgi?COMMONQUERY=LAWS). Public.leginfo.state.ny.us. . Retrieved 2012-01-09.

[10] "Sole Custody legal definition of Sole Custody. Sole Custody synonyms by the Free Online Law Dictionary" (http://legal-dictionary. thefreedictionary.com/Sole+Custody). Legal-dictionary.thefreedictionary.com. . Retrieved 2012-01-09.

[11] "Types of Child Custody" (http://www.nolo.com/article.cfm/objectId/3842C8A7-F321-45AC-B238438010EAFE24/118/246/236/ART/). Nolo.com. . Retrieved 2012-01-09.

[12] Uniform Child-Custody Jurisdiction and Enforcement Act(1997), Article 1, Section 102(3).

[13] "Child Custody Rights for Fathers | Your Child - Your Divorce" (http://yourchildyourdivorce.com/wordpress/child-custody-rights-for-fathers/). Yourchildyourdivorce.com. 2010-01-13. . Retrieved 2012-01-09.

Best_interests

Best interests or **best interests of the child** is the doctrine used by most courts to determine a wide range of issues relating to the well-being of children. The most important of these issues concern questions that arise upon the divorce or separation of the children's parents. Here are some examples:

- With whom will the children live?
- How much contact (previously termed "access" or, in some jurisdictions, "visitation") will the parents, legal guardian, or other parties be allowed (or required) to have?
- To whom and by whom will child support be paid and in what amount?

History

The use of the **best interests** doctrine represented a 20th century shift in public policy. The **best interests** doctrine is an aspect of *parens patriae,* and in the United States it has replaced the Tender Years Doctrine, which rested on the basis that children are not resilient, and almost any change in a child's living situation would be detrimental to their well-being.

Until the early 1900s, fathers were given custody of the children in case of divorce. Many U.S. states then shifted from this standard to one that completely favored the mother as the primary caregiver. In the 1970s, the Tender Years Doctrine was replaced by the best interests of the child as determined by family courts. Because many family courts continued to give great weight to the traditional role of the mother as the primary caregiver, application of this standard in custody historically tended to favor the mother of the children.

The "best interests of the child" doctrine is sometimes used in cases where non-parents, such as grandparents, ask a court to order non-parent visitation with a child. Some parents, usually those who are not awarded custody, say that using the "best interests of the child" doctrine in non-parent visitation cases fails to protect a fit parent's fundamental right to raise their child in the manner they see fit. Troxel v Granville, 530 US 57; 120 S Ct 2054; 147 LEd2d 49 (2000).

Assessing the best interests of the child

In proceedings involving divorce or the dissolution of a common-law marriage or a civil union, family courts are directed to assess the best interests of any children of these unions.

The determination is also used in proceedings which determine legal obligations and entitlements, such as when a child is born outside of marriage, when grandparents assert rights with respect to their grandchildren, and when biological parents assert rights with respect to a child who was given up for adoption.

It is the doctrine usually employed in cases regarding the potential emancipation of minors. Courts will use this doctrine when called upon to determine who should make medical decisions for a child where the parents disagree with healthcare providers or other authorities.

In determining the best interests of the child or children in the context of a separation of the parents, the court may order various investigations to be undertaken by social workers, Family Court Advisors from CAFCASS, psychologists and other forensic experts, to determine the living conditions of the child and his custodial and non-custodial parents. Such issues as the stability of the child's life, links with the community, and stability of the home environment provided by each parent may be considered by a court in deciding the child's residency in custody and visitation proceedings. In English law, section 1(1) Children Act 1989 makes the interests of any child the paramount concern of the court in all proceedings and, having indicated in s1(2) that delay is likely to prejudice the interests of any child, it requires the court to consider the "welfare checklist", i.e. the court must consider:

1. The ascertainable wishes and feelings of each child concerned (considered in light of their age and understanding)
2. Physical, emotional and/or educational needs now and in the future
3. The likely effect on any change in the circumstances now and in the future
4. Age, sex, background and any other characteristics the court considers relevant
5. Any harm suffered or at risk of suffering now and in the future
6. How capable each parent, and other person in relation to whom the court considers the question to be relevant, is of meeting the child's needs
7. The range of powers available to the court under the Children Act 1989 in the proceedings in question

The welfare checklist considers the needs, wishes and feelings of the child and young person and this analysis is vital to ensure that the human rights of children are always in the forefront of all consideration. The welfare checklist provides a comprehensive list of issues that need to be considered to ensure that young people who come into court proceedings are safeguarded fully and their rights as citizens are promoted.

Criticism of the best interests standard

The Best Interests standard has received considerable criticism by certain groups within the privacy rights and family law reform movement, particularly with regard to how it unlawfully marginalizes children from one of their parents absent a compelling government interest, and often cultivates protracted litigation. Critics argue that a higher evidentiary standard should be applied to fit parents, and that the Best Interests standard should only be applied in cases where a termination of parental rights has already occurred.

See also

- Children's rights
- Convention on the Rights of the Child

References

- Dr. Stephen Baskerville, *Taken into Custody: The War on Fathers, Marriage and the Family* Cumberland House Publishing (September 25, 2007) [1]
- Jill Elaine Hasday, *The Canon of Family Law*, Stanford Law Review, Vol. 57 (December, 2004), p. 825-900.
- Mary Ann Mason, From Father's Property To Children's Rights, A History of Child Custody [2]
- Dr. Gordon Finley, *Best interests of the child and the eye of the beholder*
- Prof. Donald Hubin, *Parental Rights and Due Process* Journal of Law & Family Studies [3]

External links

- Representing Children Worldwide [4] How Children Are Heard in Children Protective Proceedings in 250 Jurisdictions
- [5]

References

[1] http://www.amazon.com/Taken-into-Custody-Fatherhood-Marriage/dp/1581825943
[2] http://www.grad.berkeley.edu/deans/mason/booksfathersintroduction.shtml
[3] http://people.cohums.ohio-state.edu/hubin1/Research/PRDP.PDF
[4] http://www.law.yale.edu/rcw
[5] http://www.vfoc.org

Mind_control

Mind control (also known as **brainwashing, coercive persuasion, mind abuse, thought control**, or **thought reform**) refers to a process in which a group or individual "systematically uses unethically manipulative methods to persuade others to conform to the wishes of the manipulator(s), often to the detriment of the person being manipulated".[1] The term has been applied to any tactic, psychological or otherwise, which can be seen as subverting an individual's sense of control over their own thinking, behavior, emotions or decision making. In Propaganda: The Formation of Men's Attitudes, Jacques Ellul maintains that the "principal aims of these psychological methods is to destroy a man's habitual patterns, space, hours, milieu, and so on."[2]

Theories of brainwashing and of mind control were originally developed to explain how totalitarian regimes appeared to succeed in systematically indoctrinating prisoners of war through propaganda and torture techniques. These theories were later expanded and modified to explain a wider range of phenomena, especially conversions to new religious movements (NRMs).

Korean War and the origin of brainwashing

The Oxford English Dictionary records its earliest known English-language usage of *brainwashing* in an article by Edward Hunter in *New Leader* published on 7 October 1950. During the Korean War, Hunter, who worked at the time both as a journalist and as a U.S. intelligence agent, wrote a series of books and articles on the theme of Chinese brainwashing.[3]

The Chinese term (*xǐ nǎo*, literally "wash brain")[4] was originally used to describe methodologies of coercive persuasion used under the Maoist regime in China, which aimed to transform individuals with a reactionary imperialist mindset into "right-thinking" members of the new Chinese social system.[5] To that end the regime developed techniques that would break down the psychic integrity of the individual with regard to information processing, information retained in the mind and individual values. Chosen techniques included dehumanizing of individuals by keeping them in filth, sleep deprivation, partial sensory deprivation, psychological harassment, inculcation of guilt and group social pressure. The term punned on the Taoist custom of "cleansing/washing the heart/mind"[6] (, *xǐ xīn*) prior to conducting certain ceremonies or entering certain holy places.

Hunter and those who picked up the Chinese term used it to explain why, unlike in earlier wars, a relatively high percentage of American GIs defected to the enemy side after becoming prisoners-of-war. It was believed that the Chinese in North Korea used such techniques to disrupt the ability of captured troops to effectively organize and resist their imprisonment.[7] British radio operator Robert W. Ford[8] [9] and British army Colonel James Carne also claimed that the Chinese subjected them to brainwashing techniques during their war-era imprisonment. The most prominent case in the U.S. was that of Frank Schwable, who confessed to having participated in germ warfare while in captivity.[10]

After the war, two studies of the repatriation of American prisoners of war by Robert Jay Lifton[11] and by Edgar Schein[12] concluded that brainwashing (called "thought reform" by Lifton and "coercive persuasion" by Schein) had a transient effect. Both researchers found that the Chinese mainly used coercive persuasion to disrupt the ability of the prisoners to organize and maintain morale and hence to escape. By placing the prisoners under conditions of physical and social deprivation and disruption, and then by offering them more comfortable situations such as better sleeping quarters, better food, warmer clothes or blankets, the Chinese did succeed in getting some of the prisoners to make anti-American statements. Nevertheless, the majority of prisoners did not actually adopt Communist beliefs, instead behaving as though they did in order to avoid the plausible threat of extreme physical abuse. Both researchers also concluded that such coercive persuasion succeeded only on a minority of POWs, and that the end-result of such coercion remained very unstable, as most of the individuals reverted to their previous condition soon after they left the coercive environment. In 1961 they both published books expanding on these findings. Schein published

Coercive Persuasion[13] and Lifton published *Thought Reform and the Psychology of Totalism*.[14] More recent writers including Mikhail Heller have suggested that Lifton's model of brainwashing may throw light on the use of mass propaganda in other communist states such as the former Soviet Union.[15]

In a summary published in 1963, Edgar Schein gave a background history of the precursor origins of the brainwashing phenomenon:

> Thought reform contains elements which are evident in Chinese culture (emphasis on interpersonal sensitivity, learning by rote and self-cultivation); in methods of extracting confessions well known in the Papal Inquisition (13th century) and elaborated through the centuries, especially by the Russian secret police; in methods of organizing corrective prisons, mental hospitals and other institutions for producing value change; in methods used by religious sects, fraternal orders, political elites or primitive societies for converting or initiating new members. Thought reform techniques are consistent with psychological principles but were not explicitly derived from such principles.[16]

Mind-control theories from the Korean War era came under criticism in subsequent years. According to forensic psychologist Dick Anthony, the CIA invented the concept of "brainwashing" as a propaganda strategy to undercut communist claims that American POWs in Korean communist camps had voluntarily expressed sympathy for communism. Anthony stated that definitive research demonstrated that fear and duress, not brainwashing, caused western POWs to collaborate. He argued that the books of Edward Hunter (whom he identified as a secret CIA "psychological warfare specialist" passing as a journalist) pushed the CIA brainwashing theory onto the general public. He further asserted that for twenty years, starting in the early 1950s, the CIA and the Defense Department conducted secret research (notably including Project MKULTRA) in an attempt to develop practical brainwashing techniques, and that their attempt failed.[17]

The U.S. military and government laid charges of "brainwashing" in an effort to undermine detailed confessions made by U.S. military personnel to war crimes, including biological warfare, against the Koreans.[18] Frank Schwable, Chief of Staff of the First Marine Air Wing was shot down in North Korea. After Chinese radio broadcasts claimed to quote him admitting to participating in germ warfare, United Nations commander Gen. Mark W. Clark denounced said: "Whether these statements ever passed the lips of these unfortunate men is doubtful. If they did, however, too familiar are the mind-annihilating methods of these Communists in extorting whatever words they want .... The men themselves are not to blame, and they have my deepest sympathy for having been used in this abominable way."[19] In August, Secretary of Defense Charles E. Wilson set up a task force to study the response of U.S. prisoners of war to brainwashing.[20]

Army report debunks brainwashing of American prisoners of war

In 1956 the U.S Department of the Army published a report entitled <u>Communist Interrogation, Indoctrination, and Exploitation of Prisoners of War</u> which called brainwashing a "popular misconception."[21] The report states "exhaustive research of several government agencies failed to reveal even one conclusively documented case of 'brainwashing' of an American prisoner of war in Korea."[22]

While US POW's captured by North Korea were brutalized with starvation, beatings, forced death marches, exposure to extremes of temperature, binding in stress positions, and withholding of medical care, the abuse had no relation to indoctrination or collecting intelligence information "in which they [North Korea] were not particularly interested."[23] In contrast American POW's in the custody of the Chinese Communists did face a concerted interrogation and indoctrination program--but the Chinese did not employ deliberate physical abuse. "Extensive research has disclosed that systematic, physical torture was not employed in connection with interrogation or indoctrination," the report states.[24]

The Chinese elicited information using tricks such as harmless-seeming written questionnaires, followed by interviews.[25] The "most insidious" and effective Chinese technique according to the US Army Report was a convivial display of false friendship:

> "[w]hen an American soldier was captured by the Chinese, he was given a vigorous handshake and a pat on the back. The enemy 'introduced' himself as a friend of the 'workers' of America . . . in many instances the Chinese did not search the American captives, but frequently offered them American cigarettes. This display of friendship caught most Americans totally off-guard and they never recovered from the initial impression made by the Chinese. . . . [A]fter the initial contact with the enemy, some Americans seemed to believe that the enemy was sincere and harmless. They relaxed and permitted themselves to be lulled into a well-disguised trap [of cooperating with] the cunning enemy." [26]

It was this surprising, disarmingly friendly treatment, that "was successful to some degree," the report concludes, in undermining hatred of the communists among American soldiers, in persuading some to sign anti-American confessions, and even leading a few to reject repatriation and remain in Communist China.[27]

Cults and the shift of focus

After the Korean War, applications of mind control theories in the United States shifted in focus from politics to religion. From the 1960s an increasing number of American youths started to come into contact with new religious movements (NRM), and some who converted suddenly adopted beliefs and behaviors that differed greatly from those of their families and friends; in some cases they neglected or even broke contact with their loved ones. In the 1970s the anti-cult movement applied mind control theories to explain these sudden and seemingly dramatic religious conversions.[28] [29] [30] The media was quick to follow suit,[31] and social scientists sympathetic to the anti-cult movement, who were usually psychologists, developed more sophisticated models of brainwashing.[29] While some psychologists were receptive to these theories, sociologists were for the most part skeptical of their ability to explain conversion to NRMs.[32]

Theories of mind control and religious conversion

Over the years various theories of conversion and member retention have been proposed that link mind control to NRMs, and particularly those religious movements referred to as "cults" by their critics. These theories resemble the original political brainwashing theories with some minor changes. Philip Zimbardo discusses mind control as "the process by which individual or collective freedom of choice and action is compromised by agents or agencies that modify or distort perception, motivation, affect, cognition and/or behavioral outcomes",[33] and he suggests that any human being is susceptible to such manipulation.[34] In a 1999 book, Robert Lifton also applied his original ideas about thought reform to Aum Shinrikyo, concluding that in this context thought reform was possible without violence or physical coercion. Margaret Singer, who also spent time studying the political brainwashing of Korean prisoners of war, agreed with this conclusion: in her book *Cults in Our Midst* she describes six conditions which would create an atmosphere in which thought reform is possible.[35]

Approaching the subject from the perspective of neuroscience and social psychology, Kathleen Taylor suggests that manipulation of the prefrontal cortex activates "brainwashing", rendering a person more susceptible to black-and-white thinking.[36] Meanwhile, in *Influence, Science and Practice*, social psychologist Robert Cialdini argues that mind control is possible through the covert exploitation of the unconscious rules that underlie and facilitate healthy human social interactions. He states that common social rules can be used to prey upon the unwary. Using categories, he offers specific examples of both mild and extreme mind control (both one on one and in groups), notes the conditions under which each social rule is most easily exploited for false ends, and offers suggestions on how to resist such methods.[37]

Deprogramming and the anti-cult movement

Both academic and non-academic critics of "destructive cults" have adopted and adapted the theories of Singer, Lifton and other researchers from the inception of the anti-cult movement onwards. Such critics often argue that certain religious groups use mind control techniques to unethically recruit and maintain members. Many of these critics advocated or engaged in deprogramming as a method to liberate group members from apparent "brainwashing". However the practice of coercive deprogramming fell out of favor in the West and was largely superseded by exit counseling. Exit counselor Steven Hassan promotes what he calls the "BITE" model in his book *Releasing the Bonds: Empowering People to Think for Themselves* (2000).[38] The BITE model describes various controls over human behavior, information, thought and emotion.[38] Hassan claims that cults recruit and retain members by using, among other things, systematic deception, behavior modification, the withholding of information, and emotionally intense persuasion techniques (such as the induction of phobias). He refers to all of these techniques collectively as "mind control".

Critics of mind control theories caution against the broader implications of these conversion models. In the 1998 Enquete Commission report on "So-called Sects and Psychogroups" in Germany, a review was made of the BITE model. The report concluded that "control of these areas of action is an inevitable component of social interactions in a group or community. The social control that is always associated with intense commitment to a group must therefore be clearly distinguished from the exertion of intentional, methodical influence for the express purpose of manipulation."[39] Indeed virtually all of these models share the notion that converts are in fact innocent "victims" of mind-control techniques.[32] Hassan suggests that even the cult members manipulating the new converts may themselves be sincerely misled people.[40] By considering NRM members innocent "victims" of psychological coercion these theories open the door for psychological treatments.

Sociologists including Eileen Barker have criticized theories of conversion precisely because they function to justify costly interventions such as deprogramming or exit counseling.[41] For similar reasons, Barker and other scholars have criticized mental health professionals like Margaret Singer for accepting lucrative expert witness jobs in court cases involving NRMs.[41] Singer was perhaps the most publicly notable scholarly proponent of "cult" brainwashing theories, and she became the focal point of the relative demise of those same theories within her discipline.[29]

Scholarly debate

James Richardson observes that if the NRMs had access to powerful brainwashing techniques, one would expect that NRMs would have high growth rates, yet in fact most have not had notable success in recruitment. Most adherents participate for only a short time, and the success in retaining members is limited.[42] For this and other reasons, sociologists of religion including David Bromley and Anson Shupe consider the idea that "cults" are brainwashing American youth to be "implausible."[43] In addition to Bromley, Thomas Robbins, Dick Anthony, Eileen Barker, Newton Maloney, Massimo Introvigne, John Hall, Lorne Dawson, Anson Shupe, Gordon Melton, Marc Galanter, Saul Levine (amongst other scholars researching NRMs) have argued and established to the satisfaction of courts, of relevant professional associations and of scientific communities that there exists no scientific theory, generally accepted and based upon methodologically sound research, that supports the brainwashing theories as advanced by the anti-cult movement.[44]

Other scholars disagree with this consensus amongst sociologists of religion. Benjamin Zablocki asserts that it's obvious that brainwashing occurs, at least to any objective observer; the "real sociological issue", he states, is whether "brainwashing occurs frequently enough to be considered an important social problem".[45] Zablocki disagrees with scholars like Richardson, stating that Richardson's observation is flawed.[46] According to Zablocki, Richardson misunderstands brainwashing, conceiving of it as a recruiting process, instead of a retaining process.[47] So although Richardson's data are correct, Zablocki states, properly understood, brainwashing does not imply that NRMs will have a notable success in recruitment; so the criticism is inapt.[48] Additionally, Zablocki attempts to debunk the other criticisms Richardson, et al, apply to brainwashing: if Zablocki is correct, there's a plethora of evidence in favor of the claim that some NRMs brainwash some of their members.[49] Perhaps most notably, Zablocki says, the sheer number of former cult leaders and ex-members who attest to brainwashing in interviews (performed in accordance with guidelines of the National Institute of Mental Health and National Science Foundation) is too large to be a result of anything other than a genuine phenomenon.[50] Zablocki also reveals that of two most prestigious journals dedicated to the sociology of religion, the number of articles "supporting the brainwashing perspective" have been zero, while over one hundred such articles have been published in other journals "marginal to the field".[51] From this fact, Zablocki concludes that the concept 'brainwashing' has been "blacklisted" unfairly from the field of sociology of religion.[51] Moreover, sociologists of religion have received "lavish funding" from NRMs, which suggests that the so-called scientific community of scholars engages in some "corrupt" practices.[45] Stephen A. Kent has also published several articles about brainwashing.[52] [53] These scholars tend to see no consensus, while what Melton sees as a majority of scholars[54] may regard it as a rejection of brainwashing and of mind control as legitimate theories.

Legal issues, the APA and DIMPAC

Since their inception, mind control theories have also been used in various legal proceedings against "cult" groups. In 1980, ex-Scientologist Lawrence Wollersheim successfully sued the Church of Scientology in a California court which decided in 1986 that church practices had been conducted in a psychologically coercive environment and so were not protected by religious freedom guarantees. Others who have tried claiming a "brainwashing defense" for crimes committed while purportedly under mind control, including Patty Hearst, Steven Fishman and Lee Boyd Malvo, have not been successful.

In 1983, the American Psychological Association (APA) asked Margaret Singer to chair a taskforce called the APA Task Force on Deceptive and Indirect Techniques of Persuasion and Control (DIMPAC) to investigate whether brainwashing or "coercive persuasion" did indeed play a role in recruitment by such movements. Before the taskforce had submitted its final report, the APA submitted on February 10, 1987 an *amicus curiæ* brief in an ongoing court case related to brainwashing. Although the amicus curiæ brief written by the APA denies the credibility of the brainwashing theory, the APA submitted the brief under "intense pressure by a consortium of pro-religion scholars (a.k.a. NRM scholars)".[55] The brief repudiated Singer's theories on "coercive persuasion" and suggested that brainwashing theories were without empirical proof.[56] Afterward the APA filed a motion to withdraw its signature from the brief, since Singer's final report had not been completed.[57] However, on May 11, 1987, the APA's Board of Social and Ethical Responsibility for Psychology (BSERP) rejected the DIMPAC report because the report "lacks the scientific rigor and evenhanded critical approach necessary for APA imprimatur", and concluded that "after much consideration, BSERP does not believe that we have sufficient information available to guide us in taking a position on this issue."[58] This leaves the APA's position on brainwashing as equivalent to: more research is needed until a definitive scientific verdict can be given.[59]

Two critical letters from external reviewers Benjamin Beit-Hallahmi and Jeffery D. Fisher accompanied the rejection memo. The letters criticized "brainwashing" as an unrecognized theoretical concept and Singer's reasoning as so flawed that it was "almost ridiculous."[60] After her findings were rejected, Singer sued the APA in 1992 for "defamation, frauds, aiding and abetting and conspiracy" and lost.[61] Benjamin Zablocki and Alberto Amitrani interpreted the APA's response as meaning that there was no unanimous decision on the issue either way, suggesting also that Singer retained the respect of the psychological community after the incident.[62] Yet her career as an expert witness ended at this time. She was meant to appear with Richard Ofshe in the 1990 U.S. v. Fishman Case, in which Steven Fishman claimed to have been under mind control by the Church of Scientology in order to defend himself against charges of embezzlement, but the courts disallowed her testimony. In the eyes of the court, "neither the APA nor the ASA has endorsed the views of Dr. Singer and Dr. Ofshe on thought reform".[63]

After that time U.S. courts consistently rejected testimonies about mind control and manipulation, stating that such theories were not part of accepted mainline science according to the Frye Standard (Anthony & Robbins 1992: 5-29) of 1923.

Other areas

Mind control is a general term for a number of controversial theories proposing that an individual's thinking, behavior, emotions or decisions can, to a greater or lesser extent, be manipulated at will by outside sources. According to sociologist James T. Richardson, some of the concepts of brainwashing have spread to other fields and are applied "with some success" in contexts unrelated to the earlier cult controversies, such as custody battles and child sexual abuse cases, "where one parent is accused of brainwashing the child to reject the other parent, and in child sex abuse cases where one parent is accused of brainwashing the child to make sex abuse accusations against the other parent".[64] [65]

Stephen A. Kent analyzes and summarizes the use of the brainwashing meme by non-sociologists in the period 2000-2007, finding the term useful not only in the context of "New Religions/Cults", but equally under the headings of "Teen Behavior Modification Programs; Terrorist Groups; Dysfunctional Corporate Culture; Interpersonal Violence; and Alleged Chinese Governmental Human Rights Violations Against Falun Gong".[66]

See also

* APA Task Force on Deceptive and Indirect Techniques of Persuasion and Control
* Crowd manipulation
* Culture of fear
* Destabilisation
* Gaslighting
* Indoctrination
* *Jason Scott* case
* Love bombing
* Mind control in popular culture
* Mind games
* MKULTRA (a covert CIA research program)
* Propaganda, and Propaganda model
* Propaganda: The Formation of Men's Attitudes
* Subliminal messages
* Unethical human experimentation in the United States

References

[1] Langone, Michael. "Cults: Questions and Answers" (http://www.csj.org/studyindex/studycult/cultqa.htm). *www.csj.org*. International Cultic Studies Association. . Retrieved 2009-12-27. "Mind control (also referred to as 'brainwashing,' 'coercive persuasion,' 'thought reform,' and the 'systematic manipulation of psychological and social influence') refers to a process in which a group or individual systematically uses unethically manipulative methods to persuade others to conform to the wishes of the manipulator(s), often to the detriment of the person being manipulated."

[2] Ellul, Jacques (1973). *Propaganda: The Formation of Men's Attitudes*, p. 113.Trans. Konrad Kellen & Jean Lerner. Vintage Books, New York. ISBN 978-0-394-71874-3.

[3] Marks, John (1979). "8. Brainwashing" (http://www.druglibrary.org/schaffer/lsd/marks8.htm). *The Search for the Manchurian Candidate: The CIA and Mind Control* (http://www.druglibrary.org/schaffer/LSD/marks.htm). New York: Times Books. ISBN 0-8129-0773-6. . Retrieved 2008-12-30. "In September 1950, the *Miami News* published an article by Edward Hunter titled " 'Brain-Washing' Tactics Force Chinese into Ranks of Communist Party." It was the first printed use in any language of the term "brainwashing," which quickly became a stock phrase in Cold War headlines. Hunter, a CIA propaganda operator who worked under cover as a journalist, turned out a steady stream of books and articles on the subject."

[4] Chinese English Dictionary (http://www.mdbg.net/chindict/chindict.php?page=worddict&wdrst=0&wdqb=æ´è¦)

[5] Taylor, Kathleen (2006). *Brainwashing: The Science of Thought Control* (http://books.google.com/?id=D3tYeMLc4hQC). Oxford: Oxford University Press. p. 5. ISBN 9780199204786. . Retrieved 2010-07-02.

[6] **Note:** can mean "heart", "mind" or "centre" depending on context. For example, means Cardiovascular disease, but means psychologist, and means Central business district.

[7] Browning, Michael (2003-03-14). "Was Kidnapped Utah Teen Brainwashed?". *Palm Beach Post* (Palm Beach). ISSN 1528-5758. "During the Korean War, captured American soldiers were subjected to prolonged interrogations and harangues by their captors, who often worked in relays and used the "good-cop, bad-cop" approach, alternating a brutal interrogator with a gentle one. It was all part of "Xi Nao," washing the brain. The Chinese and Koreans were making valiant attempts to convert the captives to the communist way of thought."

[8] Ford RC (1990). *Captured in Tibet.* Oxford [Oxfordshire]: Oxford University Press. ISBN 0-19-581570-X.

[9] Ford RC (1997). *Wind Between the Worlds: Captured in Tibet.* SLG Books. ISBN 0-9617066-9-4.

[10] *New York Times*: "Red Germ Charges Cite 2 U.S. Marines," February 23, 1954 (http://query.nytimes.com/mem/archive/pdf?res=F40C16FC3C5A107B93C1AB1789D85F478585F9), accessed February 16, 2012

[11] Lifton, Robert J. (1954-04). "Home by Ship: Reaction Patterns of American Prisoners of War Repatriated from North Korea" (http://ajp. psychiatryonline.org/cgi/content/abstract/110/10/732). *American Journal of Psychiatry* **110** (10): 732–739. doi:10.1176/appi.ajp.110.10.732. PMID 13138750. . Retrieved 2008-03-30. Cited in *Thought Reform and the Psychology of Totalism*

[12] Schein, Edgar (1956-05). "The Chinese Indoctrination Program for Prisoners of War: A Study of Attempted Brainwashing". *Psychiatry* **19** (2): 149–172. PMID 13323141. Cited in *Thought Reform and the Psychology of Totalism*

[13] Schein, Edgar H. (1971). *Coercive Persuasion: A Socio-Psychological Analysis of the "Brainwashing" of American Civilian Prisoners by the Chinese Communists.* New York: W.W. Norton. ISBN 0-393-00613-1.

[14] Lifton, RJ (1989) [1961]. Thought Reform and the Psychology of Totalism; a Study of "Brainwashing" in China. Chapel Hill: University of North Carolina Press. ISBN 0-8078-4253-2.

[15] Heller, Mikhail (1988). Cogs in the Soviet Wheel: The Formation of Soviet Man. Translated by David Floyd. London: Collins Harvill. ISBN 0-00-272516-9. "Dr [Robert J.] Lifton draws attention to a fact of exceptional importance: the effect of 'brainwashing' and its methods is felt even by those whom he calls the 'apparent resisters', those who seem not to succumb to the intoxication. This study showed that they do assimilate what has been hammered into their brain but the effect comes only a certain time after their liberation, like the explosion of a delayed-action bomb. It is not hard to imagine the effect which 'education' and 're-education' has upon the Soviet citizen, who is exposed from the day he is born to 'brainwashing', bombarded every day, round the clock, by all the means of propaganda and persuasion." Heller's footnote explains the phrase "the means of propaganda and persuasion" as "[t]he official name for the means of communication in the USSR. The accepted abbreviation is SMIP [literally from the Russian phrase meaning 'means of mass information and propaganda']."

[16] Schein, Edgar Henry (1963). "Brainwashing". *Encyclopædia Britannica.* **4** (14th (revised) ed.). Encyclopædia Britannica, Inc.. p. 91.

[17] Anthony, Dick (1999). "Pseudoscience and Minority Religions: An Evaluation of the Brainwashing Theories of Jean-Marie". *Social Justice Research* **12** (4): 421–456. doi:10.1023/A:1022081411463.

[18] Stephen Endicott and Edward Hagerman, *The United States and Biological Warfare: Secrets From the Early Cold War* (Indiana University Press, 1998)

[19] *New York Times*: "Clark Denounces Germ War Charges," February 24, 1953 (http://query.nytimes.com/mem/archive/pdf?res=F10C10FC3D5B107A93C6AB1789D85F478585F9), accessed February 16, 2012

[20] *New York Times*: "Officers to Study 'Brainwash' Issue," August 23, 1954 (http://query.nytimes.com/mem/archive/pdf?res=F40E16F83A5A107B93C1AB1783D85F408585F9), accessed February 16, 2012

[21] U.S Department of the Army (15 May 1956). *Communist Interrogation, Indoctrination, and Exploitation of Prisoners of War.* (Pamphlet No. 30-101 ed.). U.S Gov't Printing Office. pp. 17 & 51.

[22] (Communist Interrogation, Indoctrination, and Exploitation of Prisoners of War 1956, p. 51)

[23] (Communist Interrogation, Indoctrination, and Exploitation of Prisoners of War 1956, p. 15)North Koreans considered US POWs illegal invaders and asserted they were not protected by the Geneva Conventions.

[24] (Communist Interrogation, Indoctrination, and Exploitation of Prisoners of War 1956, p. 51)

[25] (Communist Interrogation, Indoctrination, and Exploitation of Prisoners of War 1956, p. 20-21)

[26] (Communist Interrogation, Indoctrination, and Exploitation of Prisoners of War 1956, p. 37)

[27] (Communist Interrogation, Indoctrination, and Exploitation of Prisoners of War 1956, p. 50-51)

[28] Melton, J. Gordon (1999-12-10). "Brainwashing and the Cults: The Rise and Fall of a Theory" (http://www.cesnur.org/testi/melton. htm). CESNUR: Center for Studies on New Religions. . Retrieved 2009-06-15. "In the United States at the end of the 1970s, brainwashing emerged as a popular theoretical construct around which to understand what appeared to be a sudden rise of new and unfamiliar religious movements during the previous decade, especially those associated with the hippie street-people phenomenon."

[29] Bromley, David G. (1998). "Brainwashing". In William H. Swatos Jr. (Ed.). *Encyclopedia of Religion and Society.* Walnut Creek, CA: AltaMira. pp. 61–62. ISBN 978-0761989561.

[30] Barker, Eileen: *New Religious Movements: A Practical Introduction.* London: Her Majesty's Stationery office, 1989.

[31] Wright, Stewart A. (1997). "Media Coverage of Unconventional Religion: Any 'Good News' for Minority Faiths?". *Review of Religious Research* (Review of Religious Research, Vol. 39, No. 2) **39** (2): 101–115. doi:10.2307/3512176. JSTOR 3512176.

[32] Barker, Eileen (1986). "Religious Movements: Cult and Anti-Cult Since Jonestown". *Annual Review of Sociology* **12**: 329–346. doi:10.1146/annurev.so.12.080186.001553.

[33] Zimbardo, Philip G. (November 2002). "Mind Control: Psychological Reality or Mindless Rhetoric?" (http://www.icsahome.com/infoserv_articles/zimbardo_philip_mindcontrol.htm). *Monitor on Psychology*. . Retrieved 2008-12-30. "Mind control is the process by which individual or collective freedom of choice and action is compromised by agents or agencies that modify or distort perception, motivation,

affect, cognition and/or behavioral outcomes. It is neither magical nor mystical, but a process that involves a set of basic social psychological principles. Conformity, compliance, persuasion, dissonance, reactance, guilt and fear arousal, modeling and identification are some of the staple social influence ingredients well studied in psychological experiments and field studies. In some combinations, they create a powerful crucible of extreme mental and behavioral manipulation when synthesized with several other real-world factors, such as charismatic, authoritarian leaders, dominant ideologies, social isolation, physical debilitation, induced phobias, and extreme threats or promised rewards that are typically deceptively orchestrated, over an extended time period in settings where they are applied intensively. A body of social science evidence shows that when systematically practiced by state-sanctioned police, military or destructive cults, mind control can induce false confessions, create converts who willingly torture or kill 'invented enemies,' and engage indoctrinated members to work tirelessly, give up their money—and even their lives—for 'the cause.'"

[34] Zimbardo, P (1997). "What messages are behind today's cults?" (http://www.csj.org/studyindex/studycult/study_zimbar.htm). *Monitor on Psychology*: 14. .

[35] *Cults in Our Midst: The Continuing Fight Against Their Hidden Menace* (http://www.refocus.org/singerne.html), Margaret Thaler Singer, Jossey-Bass, publisher, April 2003, ISBN 0-78796-741-6

[36] Taylor, Kathleen Eleanor (December 2004). *[[Brainwashing: The Science of Thought Control* (http://books.google.com/ ?id=BIuju20yhDkC&dq)]]. Oxford University Press. p. 215. ISBN 9780192804969. . Retrieved 2009-07-30. "Your susceptibility to brainwashing (and other forms of influence) has much to do with the state of your brain. This will depend in part on your genes: research suggests that prefrontal function is substantially affected by genetics. Low educational achievement, dogmatism, stress, and other factors which affect prefrontal function encourage simplistic, black-and-white thinking. If you have neglected your neurons, failed to stimulate your synapses, obstinately resisted new experiences, or hammered your prefrontal cortex with drugs (including alcohol), lack of sleep, rollercoaster emotions, or chronic stress, you may well be susceptible to the totalist charms of the next charismatic you meet. This is why so many young people baffle their more phlegmatic elders by joining cults, developing obsessions with fashions and celebrities, and forming intense attachments to often unsuitable role models."*

[37] Cialdini, Robert B. (2007). *Influence: the psychology of persuasion*. London: Collins. pp. epilogue. ISBN 0-06-124189-X.

[38] *Releasing the Bonds: Empowering People to Think for Themselves*, Steven Hassan, Ch. 2, Aitan Publishing Company, 2000

[39] Final Report of the Enquete Commission on "So-called Sects and Psychogroups" New Religious and Ideological Communities and Psychogroups in the Federal Republic of Germany (http://www.agpf.de/Bundestag-Enquete-english.pdf)

[40] Hassan, Steven (1988). *Combatting cult mind control*. Rochester, Vt: Park Street Press. ISBN 0-89281-243-5.

[41] Barker, Eileen (1995). "The Scientific Study of Religion? You Must Be Joking!". *Journal for the Scientific Study of Religion* (Journal for the Scientific Study of Religion, Vol. 34, No. 3) **34** (3): 287–310. doi:10.2307/1386880. JSTOR 1386880.

[42] Richardson, James T. (1985-06). "The active vs. passive convert: paradigm conflict in conversion/recruitment research". *Journal for the Scientific Study of Religion* (Journal for the Scientific Study of Religion, Vol. 24, No. 2) **24** (2): 163–179. doi:10.2307/1386340. JSTOR 1386340.

[43] Brainwashing by Religious Cults (http://www.religioustolerance.org/brain_wa.htm)

[44] CESNUR - Brainwashing and Mind Control Controversies (http://www.cesnur.org/testi/gandow_eng.htm)

[45] Zablocki, Benjamin. (1997-10). "THE BLACKLISTING OF A CONCEPT: THE STRANGE HISTORY OF THE BRAINWASHING CONJECTURE IN THE SOCIOLOGY OF RELIGION". *Nova religio* **1** (1): 96-121.

[46] Zablocki, Benjamin (2001). *Misunderstanding Cults: Searching for Objectivity in a Controversial Field*. U of Toronto Press. pp. 176. ISBN 0802081886.

[47] Zablocki, Benjamin (2001). *Misunderstanding Cults: Searching for Objectivity in a Controversial Field*. U of Toronto Press. pp. 176. ISBN 0802081886.

[48] Zablocki, Benjamin (2001). *Misunderstanding Cults: Searching for Objectivity in a Controversial Field*. U of Toronto Press. pp. 176. ISBN 0802081886.

[49] Zablocki, Benjamin (2001). *Misunderstanding Cults: Searching for Objectivity in a Controversial Field*. U of Toronto Press. pp. 176. ISBN 0802081886.

[50] Zablocki, Benjamin (2001). *Misunderstanding Cults: Searching for Objectivity in a Controversial Field*. U of Toronto Press. pp. 194-201. ISBN 0802081886.

[51] Zablocki, Benjamin. (1998-04). "TReply to Bromley". *Nova religio* **1** (2): 267-271.

[52] Brainwashing and Re-Indoctrination Programs in the Children of God/The Family (http://www.nospank.net/kent.htm)

[53] Dr. Stephen A. Kent (1997-11-07) (PDF). *Brainwashing in Scientology's Rehabilitation Force (RPF)* (http://www.hamburg.de/servlet/ contentblob/109286/brainwashing-pdf/data.pdf). . Retrieved 2008-08-16.

[54] Melton, J. Gordon (10 December 1999). "Brainwashing and the Cults: The Rise and Fall of a Theory" (http://www.cesnur.org/testi/ melton.htm). CESNUR: Center for Studies on New Religions. . Retrieved 5 September 2009. "Since the late 1980s, though a significant public belief in cult-brainwashing remains, the academic community-including scholars from psychology, sociology, and religious studies-have shared an almost unanimous consensus that the coercive persuasion/brainwashing thesis proposed by Margaret Singer and her colleagues in the 1980s is without scientific merit."

[55] Zablocki, Benjamin (2001). *Misunderstanding Cults: Searching for Objectivity in a Controversial Field*. U. of Torono Press. pp. 168. ISBN 0802081886.

[56] CESNUR - APA Brief in the Molko Case. *[t]he methodology of Drs. Singer and Benson has been repudiated by the scientific community [... the hypotheses advanced by Singer comprised] little more than uninformed speculation, based on skewed data [...] [t]he coercive persuasion*

theory ... is not a meaningful scientific concept. [...] The theories of Drs. Singer and Benson are not new to the scientific community. After searching scrutiny, the scientific community has repudiated the assumptions, methodologies, and conclusions of Drs. Singer and Benson. The validity of the claim that, absent physical force or threats, "systematic manipulation of the social influences" can coercively deprive individuals of free will lacks any empirical foundation and has never been confirmed by other research. The specific methods by which Drs. Singer and Benson have arrived at their conclusions have also been rejected by all serious scholars in the field. (http://www.cesnur.org/testi/molko_brief.htm)

[57] Motion of the American Psychological Association to Withdraw as Amicus Curiae (http://www.rickross.com/reference/apologist/apologist25.html)

[58] American Psychological Association Board of Social and Ethical Responsibility for Psychology (BSERP) (1987-05-11). "Memorandum" (http://www.cesnur.org/testi/APA.htm). *CESNUR: APA Memo of 1987 with Enclosures*. CESNUR Center for Studies on New Religion. . Retrieved 2008-11-18. "BSERP thanks the Task Force on Deceptive and Indirect Methods of Persuasion and Control for its service but is unable to accept the report of the Task Force. In general, the report lacks the scientific rigor and evenhanded critical approach necessary for APA imprimatur."

[59] Zablocki, Benjamin (2001). *isunderstanding Cults: Searching for Objectivity in a Controversial Field*. U of Toronto Press. pp. 168. ISBN 0802081886.

[60] APA memo and two enclosures (http://www.cesnur.org/testi/APA.htm)

[61] Case No. 730012-8 (http://www.cesnur.org/testi/singer.htm) Margaret Singer v. American Psychological Association

[62] Amitrani, Alberto; Di Marzio R (2001). "Blind, or just don't want to see? Mind Control in New Religious Movements and the American Psychological Association" (http://www.csj.org/infoserv_articles/amitrani_alberto_apaandmindcontrol.htm). *Cultic Studies Review*. .

[63] *Brainwashed! Scholars of Cults Accuse Each Other of Bad Faith*, Lingua Franca, December 1998.

[64] Richardson, James T. *Regulating Religion: Case Studies from Around the Globe*, Kluwer Academic/Plenum Publishers 2004, p. 16, ISBN 9780306478871.

[65] Oldenburg, Don (2003-11-21). "Stressed to Kill: The Defense of Brainwashing; Sniper Suspect's Claim Triggers More Debate" (http://www.crimlaw.org/defbrief269.html), *Washington Post*, reproduced in *Defence Brief*, issue 269, published by Steven Skurka & Associates

[66] Kent, Stephen A. (2008). "Contemporary Uses of the Brainwashing Concept: 2000 to Mid-2007" (http://www.icsahome.com/logon/elibdocview_new.asp?Subject=Contemporary+Uses+of+the+Brainwashing+Concept:+2000+to+Mid-2007). *Cultic Studies Review* (International Cultic Studies Association) 7 (2): 99–128. ISSN 1539-0152. . Retrieved 2010-02-09. "The brainwashing concept is sufficiently useful that it continues to appear in a wide variety of legal, political, and social contexts. This article identifies those contexts by summarizing its appearance in court cases, discussions about cults and former cult members, terrorists, and alleged victims of state repression between the years 2000 and mid-2007. In creating this summary, we discover that a physiologist has examined the biochemical aspects of persons going through brainwashing processes, and that (to varying degrees) some judges and others related to the judiciary have realized that people who have been through these processes have impaired judgment and often need special counseling. Most dramatically, a new brainwashing program may be operating in Communist China, a country whose political activities toward its own citizens in the late 1940s and 1950s spawned so much of the initial brainwashing research."

Further reading

- Begich N (2006). *Controlling the Human Mind*. Anchorage, AK. ISBN 1-890693-54-5.
- Ellul, Jacques. *Propaganda: The Formation of Men's Attitudes*. Trans. Konrad Kellen & Jean Lerner. New York: Knopf, 1965. New York: Random House/ Vintage 1973
- Langone MD (1993). Recovery from Cults: Help for Victims of Psychological and Spiritual Abuse. New York: Norton. ISBN 0-393-31321-2.
- Lifton RJ (1989). *Thought Reform and the Psychology of Totalism: A Study of "Brainwashing" in China*. Chapel Hill: University of North Carolina Press. ISBN 0-8078-4253-2.
- Singer M et. al. (1986-11-01). "Report of the APA Task Force on Deceptive and Indirect Techniques of Persuasion and Control (DIMPAC report)" (http://www.rickross.com/reference/apologist/apologist23.html). American Psychological Association. Retrieved 2008-10-10.
- Streatfeild D (2008). *Brainwash: The Secret History of Mind Control*. New York: Picador. ISBN 0-312-42792-1.
- Zablocki, B (1997). "The Blacklisting of a Concept. The Strange History of the Brainwashing Conjecture in the Sociology of Religion". *Nova Religio* 1 (1): 96–121. doi:10.1525/nr.1997.1.1.96.
- Zablocki, B (1998). "Exit Cost Analysis: A New Approach to the Scientific Study of Brainwashing" (http://caliber.ucpress.net/doi/pdf/10.1525/nr.1998.1.2.216) (PDF). *Nova Religio* 2 (1): 216–249. doi:10.1525/nr.1998.1.2.216. Retrieved 2008-10-10.
- Zimbardo P (2002-11-01). "Mind Control: Psychological Reality or Mindless Rhetoric?" (http://www.csj.org/infoserv_articles/zimbardo_philip_mindcontrol.htm). *Monitor on Psychology*.

- Swirski, Peter (2011). " We Better Kill the Instinct to Kill Before It Kills Us or Violence, Mind Control, and Walker Percy's *The Thanatos Syndrome*". *American Utopia and Social Engineering in Literature, Social Thought, and Political History*. New York, Routledge.

Massachusetts_Supreme_Judicial_Court

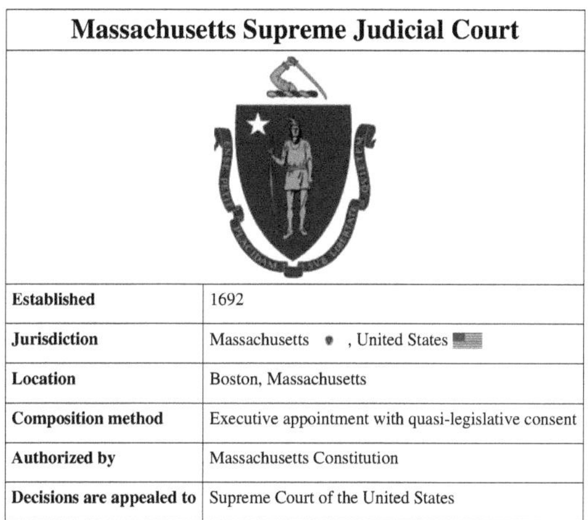

Massachusetts Supreme Judicial Court	
Established	1692
Jurisdiction	Massachusetts , United States
Location	Boston, Massachusetts
Composition method	Executive appointment with quasi-legislative consent
Authorized by	Massachusetts Constitution
Decisions are appealed to	Supreme Court of the United States

The **Massachusetts Supreme Judicial Court (SJC)** is the highest court in the Commonwealth of Massachusetts. The SJC has the distinction of being the oldest continuously functioning appellate court in the Western Hemisphere.

History

The court was established in 1692 as the "Superior Court of Judicature". It was formed by order of the British Crown in response to the large number of prosecutions stemming from the Salem Witch Trials. Its name was changed to the Supreme Judicial Court after the adoption of the Massachusetts Constitution in 1780. In 1804 an official case reporter was created to publish the court's decisions, and the first officially reported decision was *Gold v. Eddy* (1804).

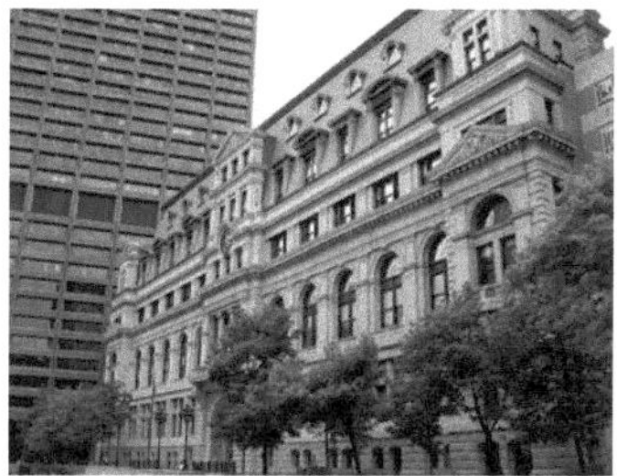

John Adams Courthouse, home to the SJC

Functions

The seven Justices hear appeals on a broad range of criminal and civil cases between September and May.

Single Justice sessions are held each week throughout the year for certain motions pertaining to cases on trial or on appeal, bail reviews, bar discipline proceedings, petitions for admission to the bar, and a variety of other statutory proceedings. The Associate Justices sit as Single Justices each month on a rotation schedule.

The full bench renders approximately 200 written decisions each year; the single justices decide a total of approximately 600 cases annually.

In addition to its appellate functions, the SJC is responsible for the general superintendence of the judiciary and of the bar, the creation or approval of rules for the operations of all the state courts, and, in certain instances, providing advisory opinions, upon request, to the Governor and General Court on various legal issues.

The SJC also has oversight responsibility in varying degrees, according to statutes, with several affiliated agencies of the judicial branch, including the Board of Bar Overseers [1], the Office of Bar Counsel [2], the Board of Bar Examiners, the Clients' Security Board, the Commission on Judicial Conduct, the Massachusetts Legal Assistance Corporation, the Massachusetts Mental Health Legal Advisors' Committee, and Correctional Legal Services, Inc.

The SJC is sits at the John Adams Courthouse, 1 Pemberton Square, Boston, Massachusetts 02108, which also houses the Massachusetts Appeals Court and the Social Law Library.

Landmark cases

- *Rex v. Preston* (1770) - Captain Thomas Preston, the Officer of the Day during the Boston Massacre, was acquitted when the jury was unable to determine whether he had ordered the troops to fire. The defense counsel in the case was a young attorney named John Adams, later the second President of the United States.

- *Rex v. Wemms, et al.* (1770) - Six soldiers involved in the Boston Massacre were found not guilty, and two more – the only two proven to have fired – were found guilty of manslaughter.

- *Commonwealth v. Nathaniel Jennison* (1783) - The Court declared slavery unconstitutional in the state of Massachusetts by allowing slaves to sue their masters for freedom. Boston lawyer, and member of the Massachusetts Constitutional Convention of 1779, John Lowell, upon the adoption of Article I for inclusion in the Massachusetts Constitution, exclaimed: *"...I will render my services as a lawyer gratis to any slave suing for his freedom if it is withheld from him..."*[3] With this case, he fulfilled his promise. Slavery in Massachusetts was denied legal standing.

- *Commonwealth v. Hunt* (1842) - The Court established that trade unions were not necessarily criminal or conspiring organizations if they did not advocate violence or illegal activities in their attempts to gain recognition through striking. This legalized the existence of non-socialist or non-violent trade organizations, though trade unions would continue to be harassed legally through anti-trust suits and injunctions.

- *Roberts v. Boston* (1850) - The Court established the "separate but equal" doctrine that would later be used in *Plessy v. Ferguson* by maintaining that the law gave school boards complete authority in assigning students to schools and that they could do so along racial lines if they deemed it appropriate.

- *Goodridge v. Department of Public Health* (2003) - The Court ruled that the denial of marriage licenses to same-sex couples violated the Massachusetts Constitution.

Composition

The Court consists of a Chief Justice and six Associate Justices appointed by the Governor of Massachusetts with the consent of the Governor's Council. The Justices hold office until the mandatory retirement age of seventy, like all other Massachusetts judges.

Current composition

The currently serving justices are:

Justice	Began active service	Appointed by
Roderick L. Ireland	1997 (Assoc.) 2010 (Chief)	William Weld (1997) Deval Patrick (2010)[4]
Margot Botsford	2007	Deval Patrick
Robert J. Cordy	2001	Paul Cellucci
Fernande R.V. Duffly	2011[5]	Deval Patrick
Ralph Gants	2009	Deval Patrick
Barbara Lenk	2011[6]	Deval Patrick
Francis X. Spina	1999	Paul Cellucci

Notable members

- William Cushing, Horace Gray, and Oliver Wendell Holmes, Jr. served on the Supreme Court of the United States after leaving the Massachusetts Supreme Judicial Court
- Charles Fried served as United States Solicitor General from 1985 to 1989 under Ronald Reagan

List of Chief Justices

Pre-Revolution

#	Chief Justice		Took office	Left office
1	William Stoughton		1692	1701
2	Wait Winthrop		1701	1701
3	Isaac Addington		1702	1703
4	Wait Winthrop		1708	1717
5	Samuel Sewall		1718	1728
6	Benjamin Lynde		1729	1745
7	Paul Dudley		1745	1751
8	Stephen Sewall		1752	1760
9	Thomas Hutchinson		1761	1769

| 10 | Benjamin Lynde | 1769 | 1771 |
| 11 | Peter Oliver | 1772 | 1775 |

Post-Revolution

#	Chief Justice		Took office	Left office
1	John Adams		1775	1776
2	William Cushing		1777	1789
3	Nathaniel Peaslee Sargent		1790	1791
4	Francis Dana		1791	1806
5	Theophilus Parsons		1806	1813
6	Samuel Sewall		1814	1814
7	Isaac Parker		August 24, 1814	July 25, 1830
8	Lemuel Shaw		August 30, 1830	August 21, 1860
9	George Tyler Bigelow		September 7, 1860	December 31, 1867
10	Reuben Atwater Chapman		February 7, 1868	June 28, 1873
11	Horace Gray		September 5, 1873	January 9, 1882
12	Marcus Morton		January 16, 1882	August 27, 1890
13	Walbridge A. Field		September 4, 1890	July 15, 1899
14	Oliver Wendell Holmes, Jr.		August 2, 1899	December 8, 1902
15	Marcus Perrin Knowlton		December 17, 1902	September 7, 1911
16	Arthur Prentice Rugg		September 20, 1911	June 12, 1938
17	Fred Tarbell Field		June 30, 1938	July 24, 1947
18	Stanley Elroy Qua		August 6, 1947	September 6, 1956
19	Raymond Sanger Wilkins		September 13, 1956	September 1, 1970
20	G. Joseph Tauro		1970	January 10, 1976
21	Edward F. Hennessey		1976	April 19, 1989
22	Paul J. Liacos		June 20, 1989	September 30, 1996
23	Herbert P. Wilkins		October 1, 1996	August 31, 1999

24	Margaret H. Marshall		October 14, 1999	December 19, 2010[7]
25	Roderick L. Ireland		December 20, 2010	Incumbent (faces mandatory retirement on December 3, 2014)

All members after 1800

Justice	Began active service	Ended active service	Appointed by
Ruth Abrams	1978	2000	Michael Dukakis
William Allen	1881	1891	John Davis Long
Charles Allen	1882	1898	John D. Long
Seth Ames	1869	1881	William Claflin
James Barker	1891	1905	William E. Russell
George Bigelow	1850	1860	George N. Briggs
Margot Botsford	2007	-	Deval Patrick
Henry Braley	1902	1929	Winthrop M. Crane
Robert Braucher	1971	1981	Francis W. Sargent
James Carroll	1915	1932	David I. Walsh
Reuben Chapman	1860	1866	Nathaniel Prentice Banks
Waldo Colburn	1882	1885	John Davis Long
James Colt	1865	1881	John Albion Andrew
Robert J. Cordy	2001	-	Paul Cellucci
Edward Counihan	1949	1960	Paul A. Dever
Judith A. Cowin	1999	2011	Paul Cellucci
Louis Cox	1937	1944	Charles F. Hurley
John C. Crosby	1914	1937	David I. Walsh
Caleb Cushing	1852	1853	George S. Boutwell
R. Ammi Cutter	1956	1972	Christian Herter
Francis Dana	1791	1806	John Hancock
Thomas Dawes	1792	1802	John Hancock
Charles Decourcy	1911	1924	Eugene Foss
Charles Devens	1873 1881	1877	William B. Washburn John D. Long
Daniel Dewey	1814	1815	Caleb Strong
Arthur Dolan	1937	1949	Charles F. Hurley
Charles Donahue	1932	1944	Joseph B. Ely
Fernande R.V. Duffly	2011	-	Deval Patrick
William Endicott	1873	1882	William B. Washburn
Fred T. Field	1929	1947	Frank G. Allen, Associate/Charles F. Hurley, Chief

Walbridge A. Field	1881	1890	John D. Long
Richard Fletcher	1848	1853	George N. Briggs
Charles Forbes	1848	1848	George N. Briggs
Dwight Foster	1866	1869	Alexander H. Bullock
Charles Fried	1995	1999	William Weld
Ralph D. Gants	2009	-	Deval Patrick
William Gardner	1885	1887	George D. Robinson
Horace Gray	1864	1881	John Albion Andrew
John M. Greaney	1989	2008	Michael Dukakis
John Hammond	1898	1914	Roger Wolcott
Edward F. Hennessey	1971	1989	Francis W. Sargent, Associate/Michael Dukakis, Chief
Ebenezer R. Hoar	1859	1869	Nathaniel Prentice Banks
Oliver Wendell Holmes, Jr.	1882	1902	John Davis Long/Associate, Roger Wolcott/Chief
Samuel Hubbard	1842	1848	John Davis
Roderick L. Ireland	1997	-	William Weld, Associate/Deval Patrick, Chief
Charles Jackson	1813	1823	Caleb Strong
Charles Jenney	1919	1923	Calvin Coolidge
Benjamin Kaplan	1972	1981	Francis W. Sargent
Paul G. Kirk, Sr.	1960	1971	Foster Furcolo
Marcus Perrin Knowlton	1887	1902	Oliver Ames
John Lathrop	1891	1906	William Russell
Barbara Lenk	2011	-	Deval Patrick
Paul J. Liacos	1976	1996	Michael Dukakis, Associate and Chief
Levi Lincoln, Sr.	1824	1825	William Eustis
Otis Lord	1875	1882	William Gaston
William Loring	1899	1919	Roger Wolcott
Henry Lummus	1932	1955	Joseph B. Ely
Neil L. Lynch	1981	2000	Edward J. King
Margaret H. Marshall	1996	2010	William Weld, Associate/Paul Cellucci, Chief
Pliny Merrick	1853	1864	John H. Clifford
Theron Metcalf	1848	1865	George N. Briggs
Marcus Morton	1825	1840	Levi Lincoln, Jr.
Marcus Morton	1869	1890	William Claflin, Associate/John Davis Long, Chief
James Morton	1890	1913	John Q. A. Brackett
Joseph Nolan	1981	1995	Edward J. King
Isaac Parker	1806	1830	Caleb Strong, Associate and Chief
Theophilus Parsons	1806	1814	Caleb Strong
Francis Patrick O'Connor	1981	1997	Edward J. King
Edward Pierce	1914	1937	Caleb Strong

Samuel Putnam	1814	1842	Caleb Strong
Stanley Qua	1934	1956	Joseph B. Ely, Associate/Robert F. Bradford, Chief
Francis Quirico	1969	1981	Francis W. Sargent
Paul Reardon	1962	1977	John A. Volpe
James Ronan	1938	1960	Charles F. Hurley
Arthur Rugg	1906	1911	Curtis Guild, Jr.
George Sanderson	1924	1932	Channing H. Cox
Theodore Sedgwick	1802	1813	Caleb Strong
Samuel Sewall	1800	1814	Caleb Strong
Lemuel Shaw	1830	1860	Levi Lincoln, Jr.
Henry Sheldon	1905	1915	William Lewis Douglas
Martha B. Sosman	2000	2007	Paul Cellucci
August Soule	1877	1881	Alexander H. Rice
John Spalding	1944	1971	Leverett Saltonstall
Jacob Spiegel	1960	1972	Foster Furcolo
Francis X. Spina	1999	-	Paul Cellucci
Simeon Strong	1801	1805	Caleb Strong
G. Joseph Tauro	1970	1976	Francis W. Sargent
George Thatcher	1801	1824	Caleb Strong
Benjamin Thomas	1853	1859	John H. Clifford
William Wait	1923	1934	Channing H. Cox
John Wells	1866	1875	Alexander H. Bullock
Arthur Whittemore	1955	1969	Christian Herter
Samuel Wilde	1815	1850	Caleb Strong
Herbert P. Wilkins	1972	1999	Francis W. Sargent, Associate/William Weld, Chief
Raymond Wilkins	1944	1970	Leverett Saltonstall, Associate/Christian Herter, Chief
Harold P. Williams	1947	1962	Robert F. Bradford

Citation

The proper legal citation for the Massachusetts Supreme Judicial Court is "Mass."

References

[1] http://www.mass.gov/obcbbo/

[2] http://www.mass.gov/obcbbo/obc.htm/

[3] Lowell, Delmar R., *The Historic Genealogy of the Lowells of America from 1639 to 1899* (p 35); Rutland VT, The Tuttle Company, 1899; ISBN 9780788415678.

[4] *Boston Globe*: Frank Phillips, "Patrick to name first African-American chief justice of SJC," November 4, 2010 (http://www.boston.com/yourtown/news/cambridge/2010/11/patrick_to_name_first_african-.html), accessed April 4, 2011

[5] *Boston Herald*: "Newest Mass. SJC Justice 'Nan' Duffly takes seat," February 7, 2011 (http://news.bostonherald.com/news/regional/view/20110207newest_mass_sjc_justice_nan_duffly_takes_seat/), accessed April 4, 2011

[6] Levenson, Michael (May 4, 2011). "Lenk approved for SJC; first openly gay justice on state's highest court" (http://www.boston.com/news/local/breaking_news/2011/05/lenk_approved_f.html). *Boston Globe*. . Retrieved May 4, 2011.

[7] *Boston Globe*: "Margaret Marshall, author of Mass. gay marriage decision, to retire," July 21, 2010 (http://www.boston.com/news/local/ breaking_news/2010/07/_the_listing_of.html), accessed April 4, 2011

External links

- Supreme Judicial Court of Massachusetts (http://www.state.ma.us/courts/courtsandjudges/courts/ supremejudicialcourt/)
- List of Chief Justices of the Supreme Judicial Court (http://www.massreports.com/justices/ChiefJustices. aspx)
- Supreme Judicial Court, Office of the Reporter of Decisions (http://www.massreports.com/)

Resources

- About the Supreme Court (http://www.state.ma.us/courts/courtsandjudges/courts/supremejudicialcourt/ about.html)
- Supreme Judicial Court Historical Society (http://www.sjchs-history.org/)
- Gay-Marriage Decision: Just the Beginning of the Debate (http://www.h-net.org/~hns/articles/2003/112903a. html)
- Memoirs v. Massachusetts (http://www.oyez.org/oyez/resource/case/239/)
- Simpson's Contemporary Quotations (http://www.bartleby.com/63/93/1793.html)

Sabotage

Sabotage, a form of political warfare, varies from highly technical *coup de main* acts that require detailed planning and the use of specially trained operatives, to innumerable simple acts which the ordinary individual citizen-saboteur can perform. Simple sabotage is carried out in such a way as to involve a minimum danger of injury, detection, and reprisal. There are two main methods of sabotage; physical destruction and the "human element." While physical destruction as a method is self-explanatory, its targets are nuanced, reflecting objects to which the saboteur has normal and inconspicuous access in everyday life. The "human element" is based on universal opportunities to make faulty decisions, to adopt a non-cooperative attitude, and to induce others to follow suit. [1]

Sabotage training for the Allies of World War II consisted of teaching would-be saboteurs the key components to working machinery on which to focus their destruction. "Saboteurs learned hundreds of small tricks to cause the Germans big trouble. The cables in a telephone junction box... could be jumbled to make the wrong connections when numbers were dialed. A few ounces of plastique, properly placed, could bring down a bridge, cave in a mine shaft, or collapse the roof of a railroad tunnel." [2]

In a workplace setting, sabotage is the conscious withdrawal of efficiency generally directed at causing some change in workplace conditions. One who engages in sabotage is a saboteur. As a rule, saboteurs try to conceal their identities because of the consequences of their actions. For example, whereas an environmental pressure group might be happy to be identified with an act of sabotage, it would not want the individual identities of the perpetrators known.

Forms of Sabotage

Acts of sabotage can be broken into several forms; both passive and active, and further by target. The forms are listed in order with the most frequently used form first:

Forms of Passive Sabotage

- Intentional loss/theft of material
- Deliberate work slowdowns/ inefficiencies
- Deliberate poor quality control of materials made
- Spoiling perishables
- Giving false directions/ false roadblocks
- Turning/ removing road signs

Forms of Active Sabotage

Used against land-based targets:

- Use of explosives
- Cutting power/ communication lines
- Mining of roads
- Arson (used along and in conjunction with attempts to sabotage fire fighting capability)
- Use of natural resources for obstacles
- Destruction or theft of livestock/crops
- Sniping
- Damaging tires
- Mining areas to prevent repair
- Fuel contamination
- Overt food/water contamination
- Covert mixing of explosives with standard fuels
- Sabotage by deception (ex: laying fake mines) with possible association of other methods of destruction
- Reduction of vehicle traction

Used against Aquatic Targets

- Water mining
- Use of underwater demolitions (swimmer saboteur)
- Sinking of obstacles in narrow passages (sometimes used in conjunction with mining)
- Running ships aground
- Arson
- Tampering (ex: opening a ship's seacocks to flood it)[3]

Types of Targets

Targets of sabotage include enemy personnel; munitions, fuels, supplies and repair facilities; aquatic targets; land routes, vehicles and weapons; industrial and economic utilities; barracks; and civil buildings. Munitions, Fuels, Supplies, and Repair Facilities as Targets of Sabotage:

- Munitions and fuel (both depots and manufacturing facilities)
- Supply depots/ warehouses
- Repair facilities
- Oil pipelines

Aquatic Targets of Sabotage:

- Ships (combatant and supply/transport)
- Water routes (canals, river, etc.)
- Harbors, piers, and docks (both from water and land routes)

Land Routes, Vehicles, and Weapons as Targets of Sabotage:

- Railways (track, switching units, etc.) and rail bridges and tunnels
- Trains (locomotive, freight, and passenger cars)
- Roads and road bridges and tunnels
- Vehicles (trucks, armored vehicles, tanks) both stationary and moving)
- Aircraft on the ground
- Artillery

Industrial and Economic Targets of Sabotage:

- Industries (both from insiders and external sabotage)
- Machinery (as opposed to an entire factory)
- Economic crops (ex: rubber tree plantations)
- Coal mines

Utilities as Targets of Sabotage:

- Communications (lines above and below ground, radar installations, radio facilities)
- Electrical facilities
- Water facilities

Barracks and Civic Buildings as Targets of Sabotage:

- Administrative and police buildings
- Troop barracks[4]

Types of Potential Saboteurs

- Terrorists or revolutionary groups
- Enemy agents
- Co-opted allied personnel
- Organized undergrounds
- Guerrilla forces
- Local sympathizers
- Special military forces[5]

Etymology

Claimed explanations include:

- That it derives from the Netherlands in the 15th century when workers would throw their sabots (wooden shoes) into the wooden gears of the textile looms to break the cogs, fearing the automated machines would render the human workers obsolete.[6]
- That it derives from the French *sabot* (a wooden shoe or clog) via its derivative *saboter* (to knock with the foot, or work carelessly).[7]
- That it derives from the late 19th-century French slang use of the word *sabot* to describe an unskilled worker, so called due to their wooden clogs or sabots; *sabotage* was used to describe the poor quality work which such workers turned out.[8]

Luddites and radical labor unions such as the Industrial Workers of the World (IWW) have advocated sabotage as a means of self-defense and direct action against unfair working conditions.

The IWW was shaped in part by the industrial unionism philosophy of Big Bill Haywood, and in 1910 Haywood was exposed to sabotage while touring Europe:

> The experience that had the most lasting impact on Haywood was witnessing a general strike on the French railroads. Tired of waiting for parliament to act on their demands, railroad workers walked off their jobs all across the country. The French government responded by drafting the strikers into the army and then ordering them back to work. Undaunted, the workers carried their strike to the job. Suddenly, they could not seem to do anything right. Perishables sat for weeks, sidetracked and forgotten. Freight bound for Paris was misdirected to Lyon or Marseille instead. This tactic — the French called it "sabotage" — won the strikers their demands and impressed Bill Haywood.[9] [10]

For the IWW, sabotage came to mean any withdrawal of efficiency — including the slowdown, the strike, or creative bungling of job assignments.[11]

One of the most severe examples was at the construction site of the Robert-Bourassa Generating Station in 1974, when workers used bulldozers to topple electric generators, damaged fuel tanks, and set buildings on fire. The project was delayed a year, and the direct cost of the damage estimated at $2 million CAD. The causes were not clear, however three factors have been cited: inter-union rivalry, poor working conditions, and the perceived arrogance of American executives of the contractor, Bechtel Corporation.[12]

As environmental action

Certain groups turn to destruction of property in order to immediately stop environmental destruction or to make visible arguments against forms of modern technology they consider detrimental to the earth and its inhabitants. The FBI and other law enforcement agencies use the term eco-terrorist when applied to damage of property. Proponents argue that since property can not feel terror, damage to property is more accurately described as sabotage. Opponents, by contrast, point out that property owners and operators can indeed feel terror. The image of the monkey wrench thrown into the moving parts of a machine to stop it from working was popularized by Edward Abbey in the novel The Monkeywrench Gang and has been adopted by eco-activists to describe destruction of earth damaging machinery.

As war tactic

In war, the word is used to describe the activity of an individual or group not associated with the military of the parties at war (such as a foreign agent or an indigenous supporter), in particular when actions result in the destruction or damaging of a productive or vital facility, such as equipment, factories, dams, public services, storage plants or logistic routes. Prime examples of such sabotage are the events of Black Tom and the Kingsland Explosion. Unlike acts of terrorism, acts of sabotage do not always have a primary objective of inflicting casualties. Saboteurs are usually classified as enemies, and like spies may be liable to prosecution and criminal penalties instead of detention as a prisoner of war. It is common for a government in power during war or supporters of the war policy to use the term loosely against opponents of the war. Similarly, German nationalists spoke of a stab in the back having cost them the loss of World War I.[13]

A modern form of sabotage is the distribution of software intended to damage specific industrial systems. For example, the CIA is alleged to have sabotaged a Siberian pipeline during the Cold War, using information from the Farewell Dossier. A more recent case may be the Stuxnet computer worm, which was designed to subtly infect and damage specific types of industrial equipment. Based on the equipment targeted and the location of infected machines, security experts believe it to be an attack on the Iranian nuclear program by the United States, Israel or, according to the latest news, even Russia.[14]

Sabotage, done well, is inherently difficult to detect and difficult to trace to its origin. During WWII, the FBI investigated 19,649 cases of sabotage and concluded the enemy had not caused any of them. [2]

There are many examples of physical sabotage in wartime. However, one of the most effective uses of sabotage is against organizations. The OSS manual provides numerous techniques under the title "General Interference with Organizations and Production":

- When possible, refer all matters to committees for "further study and consideration." Attempt to make the committees as large as possible- never less than five
- Bring up irrelevant issues as frequently as possible
- Haggle over precise wordings of communications, minutes, resolutions
- In making work assignments, always sign out the unimportant jobs first. See that the important jobs are assigned to inefficient workers of poor machines
- Insist on perfect work in relatively unimportant products; send back for refinishing those which have the least flaw. Approve other defective parts whose flaws are not visible to the naked eye
- To lower morale and with it, production, be pleasant to inefficient workers; give them undeserved promotions. Discriminate against efficient workers; complain unjustly about their work
- Hold conferences when there is more critical work to be done
- Multiply the procedures and clearances involved in issuing instructions, pay checks, and so on. See that three people have to approve everything where one would do.
- Spread disturbing rumors that sound like inside dope.

From the section entitled, "General Devices for Lowering Morale and Creating Confusion" comes the following quintessential simple sabotage advice: Act stupid. [15]

Value of Simple Sabotage in Wartime

The United States Office of Strategic Services, later renamed the CIA, noted specific value in committing simple sabotage against the enemy during wartime: "slashing tires, draining fuel tanks, starting fires, starting arguments, acting stupidly, short-circuiting electric systems, abrading machine parts will waste materials, mapower, and time." To underline the importance of simple sabotage on a widespread scale, they wrote, "widespread practice of simple sabotage will harass and demoralize enemy administrators and police." The OSS was also focused on the battle for hearts and minds during wartime; "the very practice of simple sabotage by natives in enemy or occupied territory may make these individuals identify themselves actively with the United Nations War effort, and encourage them to assist openly in periods of Allied invasion and occupation." [16]

Sabotage in the Bible

When Israel was conquered by Syria, Judas Maccabaeus led an uprising against the oppressor. Using sabotage, ambushes, and hit-and-run raid, he kept the enemy off balance, unable to use its full power against the rebels.[2]

Sabotage in World War I

On 11 January 1917, Fiodore Wozniak, using a rag saturated with phosphorous or an incendiary pencil supplied by German sabotage agents, set fire to his workbench at an ammunition assembly plant near Kingsland, NY, causing a four-hour fire that destroyed half a million 3-inch explosive shells and destroyed the plant for an estimated at 17 million in damages. Wozniak's involvement was not discovered until 1927.[17]

12 February 1917, Beduins loyal to the British destroyed a Turkish railroad near the port of Wajh, derailing a Turkish locomotive. The Beduins traveled by camel and used explosives which demolished a portion of the track.[18]

30 July 1916 Black Tom explosion

Post World War I

In Ireland, The Irish Republican Army used sabotage against the British following the Easter 1916 uprising. The IRA compromised communication lines and lines of transportation and fuel supplies. The IRA also employed passive sabotage, refusing dock and train workers to work on ships and rail cars used by the government. In 1920, agents of the IRA committed arson against at least fifteen British warehouses in Liverpool. The following year, the IRA set fire to numerous British targets again, including the Dublin Customs House, this time sabotaging most of Liverpool's firetrucks in the firehouses before lighting the matches.[19]

Sabotage in World War II

The French Resistance ran an extremely effective sabotage campaign against the Germans during WWII. Receiving their sabotage orders through messages over the BBC radio or by aircraft, the French used both passive and active forms of sabotage. Passive forms included losing German shipments and allowing poor quality material to pass factory inspections. Many active sabotage attempts were against critical rail lines of transportation. German records count 1,429 instances of sabotage from French Resistance forces between January 1942 and February 1943. From January through March 1944, sabotage accounted for three times the number of locomotives damaged by Allied airpower.[20] See also Normandy Landings for more information about sabotage on D Day.

During WWII, the Allies committed sabotage against the Peugot truck factory. After repeated failures in Allied bombing attempts to hit the factory, a team of French Resistance fighters and SOE agents distracted the German guards with a game of soccer while part of their team entered the plant and destroyed machinery.[2]

In 1944 the Germans ran a false flag sabotage infiltration, Operation Grief.

Sabotage Post WWII

From 1948-1960 the Malayan Communists committed numerous effective acts of sabotage against the Malaysian Government, first targeting railway bridges, then hitting larger targets such as military camps. Most of their efforts were centered around crippling Malaysia's economy and involved sabotage against trains, rubber trees, water pipes, and electric lines. The Communist's sabotage efforts were so successful that they caused backlash amongst the Malaysian population, who gradually withdrew support for the Communist movement as their livelihoods became threatened.[21]

In newly formed Israel from 1945-1948, Jewish groups opposed British control over Israel. Though that control was to end according to the Balfour Declaration in 1948, the groups used sabotage as an opposition tactic. The Haganah focused their efforts on camps used by the British to hold refugees and radar installations that could be used to detect illegal immigrant ships. The Stern Gang and the Irgun used terrorism and sabotage against the British government and against lines of communications. In November 1946, the Irgun and Stern Gang attacked a railroad twenty-one times in a three week period, eventually causing shell-shocked Arab railway workers to strike. The 6th Airborne Division was called in to provide security as a means of ending the strike.[22]

Sabotage in Vietnam

The Viet Cong used swimmer saboteurs often and effectively during the Vietnam War. Between 1969 and 1970, swimmers saboteurs sunk, destroyed, or damaged 77 friendly assets. Viet Cong swimmers were poorly equipped but well trained and resourceful. The swimmers provided a low cost/ low risk option with high payoff; possible loss to the country for failure compared to the possible gains from a successful mission led to the obvious conclusion the swimmer saboteurs were a good idea.[23]

Sabotage during the Cold War

On 1 January 1984, the Cuscatlan bridge over Lempa river in El Salvador, critical to flow of commercial and military traffic, was destroyed by guerilla forces using explosives after using mortar fire to "scatter" the bridge's guards, causing an estimated 3.7 million dollars in required repairs, and considerably impacted El Salvadoran business and security.[17]

In 1982 in Honduras, a group of nine Salvadorans and Nicaraguans destroyed a main electrical power station, leaving Tegucigalpa, the capital city, for three days without power. [17]

As crime

Some criminals have engaged in acts of sabotage for reasons of extortion. For example, Klaus-Peter Sabotta sabotaged German railway lines in the late 1990s in an attempt to extort DM10 million from the German railway operator Deutsche Bahn. He is now serving a sentence of life imprisonment.

As political action

Sabotage in a Coup d'Etat

Sabotage is a crucial tool of the successful coup d'etat, which requires control of communications before, during, and after the coup is staged. Simple sabotage against physical communications platforms using semi-skilled technicians, or even those trained only for this task, could effectively silence the target government of the coup, leaving the information battle space open to the dominance of the coup's leaders. To underscore the effectiveness of sabotage, "a single cooperative technician will be able temporarily to put out of action a radio station which would otherwise require a full-scale assault." [24]

Railroads, where strategically important to the regime the coup is against, are prime targets for sabotage- if a section of the track is damaged entire portions of the transportation network can be stopped until it is fixed. [25]

The term political sabotage is sometimes used to define the acts of one political camp to disrupt, harass or damage the reputation of a political opponent, usually during an electoral campaign. See Watergate.

Derivative usages

Sabotage Radio

A **sabotage radio** was a small two-way radio designed for use by resistance movements in World War II, and after the war often used by expeditions and similar parties.

Cybotage

Arquilla and Rondfeldt, in their work entitled *Networks and Netwars*, differentiate their definition of "netwar" from a list of "trendy synonyms," including "cybotage," an agglutination of the words "sabotage" and "cyber." They dub the practitioners of cybotage "cyboteurs" and note while all cybotage is not netwar, some netwar is cybotage.[26]

Counter-sabotage

Counter-sabotage, defined by Webster's dictionary, is "counterintelligence designed to detect and counteract sabotage." The United States Department of Defense definition, found in the Dictionary of Military and Associated Terms, is "Action designed to detect and counteract sabotage. See also counterintelligence"

Counter Sabotage in WWII

During WWII, British subject Eddie Chapman, trained by the Germans in sabotage, became a double agent for the British. The German Abwehr entrusted Chapman to destroy the British de Haviland Company's main plant for the manufacture of heavy bombers, but required photographic proof from their agent to verify the mission's completion. A special unit of the Royal Engineers known as the Magic Gang covered the de Haviland plant with canvas panels and scattered paper mache furniture and chunks of masonry around three broken and burnt giant generators. Photos of the plant taken from the air reflected devastation for the factory and a successful sabotage mission, and Chapman, as a British sabotage double-agent, fooled the Germans for the duration of the war.[27]

See also

- Birth control sabotage
- Edmund Charaszkiewicz
- CIA
- Cichociemni
- Colin Gubbins
- Direct action
- Espionage
- Fifth column
- Guerrilla warfare
- Industrial espionage
- Kedyw
- The Mole (TV series)
- Norwegian heavy water sabotage
- Partisan
- Political Warfare
- Setting up to fail
- Social undermining
- Special Activities Division
- Special Operations Executive
- Tampering

- Terrorism

References

[1] "Office of Strategic Services Simple Sabotage Manuel" (http://www.gutenberg.org/files/26184/page-images/26184-images.pdf). 17 January 1944. p. 1–2. . Retrieved 24 March 2012.

[2] Marrin, Albert (1985). *The Secret Armies : Spies, Counterspies, and Saboteurs in World War II*. New York: Atheneum. p. 77. ISBN 0-689-31165-6.

[3] Howard L. Douthit III, Captain, USAF (1988). *The Use and Effectiveness of Sabotage as a Means of Unconventional Warfare- An Historical Perspective from World War I Through Vietnam*. Wright-Patterson Air Force Base, Ohio: Air Force Institute of Technology.

[4] Howard L. Douthit III, Captain, USAF (1988). *The Use and Effectiveness of Sabotage as a Means of Unconventional Warfare- An Historical Perspective from World War I Through Vietnam*. Wright-Patterson Air Force Base, Ohio: Air Force Institute of Technology.

[5] Weaver, Richard L. Maj (1982). *Countersabotage: The AFOSI Role in Air Base Defense (FOUO)*. Student Report. Report No. 82-2625. Maxwell AFB AL: Air Command Staff College.

[6] Hodson, Randy and Teresa A. Sullivan, The Social Organization of Work, Chap. 3 pg. 69

[7] Partridge, Eric (1977). *Origins: A Short Etymological Dictionary of Modern English*. Routledge. p. 2843. ISBN 0203421140.

[8] Donald, Graeme (2008). *Sticklers, Sideburns & Bikinis: The Military Origins of Everyday Words and Phrases*. Osprey Publishing. p. 230. ISBN 1846033004.

[9] Roughneck, The Life and Times of Big Bill Haywood, Peter Carlson, 1983, page 152.

[10] Jimthor, Stablewars, May 2008

[11] Roughneck, The Life and Times of Big Bill Haywood, Peter Carlson, 1983, pages 196-197.

[12] Rinehart, J.W. *The Tyranny of Work*, Canadian Social Problems Series. Academic Press Canada (1975), pp. 78-79. ISBN 0-7747-3029-3.

[13] Dokumentarfilm.com (http://www.dokumentarfilm.com/en/030303.htm)

[14] Markoff, John, " Malware Aimed at Iran Hit Five Sites, Report Says (http://www.nytimes.com/2011/02/13/science/13stuxnet. html?scp=1&sq=Malware Aimed At Iran Hit Five Sites, Report Says&st=cse)", *New York Times*, 13 February 2011, p. 15.

[15] "Office of Strategic Services Simple Sabotage Manuel" (http://www.gutenberg.org/files/26184/page-images/26184-images.pdf). 17 January 1944. p. 28-31. . Retrieved 24 March 2012.

[16] "Office of Strategic Services" (http://www.gutenberg.org/files/26184/page-images/26184-images.pdf). 17 January 1944. p. 2. . Retrieved 24 March 2012.

[17] McGeorge II, Harvey J.; Christine C. Ketchem (1983–1984). "Sabotage: A Strategic Tool for Guerilla Forces". *World Affairs* (World Affairs Institute) **146** (3): 249–256. JSTOR 20671989.

[18] Conduit, D.M., et al. (1968). *Challenge and Response in Internal Conflict, Volume II: The Experience in Europe and the Middle East*. Washington: The American University.

[19] Howard L. Douthit III, Captain, USAF (1988). *The Use and Effectiveness of Sabotage as a Means of Unconventional Warfare- An Historical Perspective from World War I Through Vietnam*. Wright-Patterson Air Force Base, Ohio: Air Force Institute of Technology.

[20] Howard L. Douthit III, Captain, USAF (1988). *The Use and Effectiveness of Sabotage as a Means of Unconventional Warfare- An Historical Perspective from World War I Through Vietnam*. Wright-Patterson Air Force Base, Ohio: Air Force Institute of Technology.

[21] Report prepared by the Historical Evaluation and Research Organization under contract for the Army Research Office (1966). *Isolating the Guerrilla: Classic and Basic Case Studies (Volume II)*. Washington: Historical Evaluation and Research Organization.

[22] Conduit, D.M., et al (1967). *Challenge and Response In Internal Conflict, Volume II: The Experience in Europe and the Middle East.*. Washington: The American University.

[23] Babyak, E.E., Jr., LtJG, USN (1971). *Swimmer Sabotage or The Most Dangerous Mine*. Charleston: Naval Mine Warfare School.

[24] Luttwak, Edward (1968). *Coup d'Etat, a Practical Handbook*. London: The Penguin Press. p. 119. ISBN 0-674-17547-6.

[25] Luttwak, Edward (1968). *Coup d'Etat, a Practical Handbook*. London: The Penguin Press. p. 128. ISBN 0-674-17547-6.

[26] John Arquilla and David Ronfeldt, ed. (2001). *Networks and Netwars*. RAND. p. 5-7. ISBN 0-8330-3030-2.

[27] Marrin, Albert (1985). *The Secret Armies*. New York: Atheneum. p. 24. ISBN 0-689-31165-6.

- Émile Pouget, *Le sabotage; notes et postface de Grégoire Chamayou et Mathieu Triclot*, 1913; Mille et une nuit, 2004; English translation, *Sabotage*, paperback, 112 pp., University Press of the Pacific, 2001, ISBN 0-89875-459-3.

- Pasquinelli, Matteo. "The Ideology of Free Culture and the Grammar of Sabotage" (http://matteopasquinelli. com/docs/ideology-of-free-culture.pdf); now in *Animal Spirits: A Bestiary of the Commons*, Rotterdam: NAi Publishers, 2008.

External links

- Office of Strategic Services Simple Sabotage Manual (http://www.gutenberg.org/files/26184/page-images/26184-images.pdf)
- News, accounts and articles on workplace sabotage and organising (http://libcom.org/tags/sabotage) - Sabotage, employee theft, strikes, etc.
- Ozymandias Sabotage Handbook (http://www.reachoutpub.com/osh/)
- Ecodefense: A Field Guide to Monkeywrenching (http://theanarchistlibrary.org/HTML/Various_Authors__Ecodefense__A_Field_Guide_to_Monkeywrenching.html)
- Article on malicious railroad sabotage (http://www.du.edu/~jcalvert/railway/malice.htm)
- Elizabeth Gurley Flinn, Sabotage, the conscious withdrawal of the workers' industrial efficiency (http://www.iww.org/culture/library/sabotage/)

Parental_alienation_syndrome

Parental alienation syndrome (abbreviated as **PAS**) is term coined by Richard A. Gardner in the early 1980s to refer to what he describes as a disorder in which a child, on an ongoing basis, belittles and insults one parent without justification, due to a combination of factors, including indoctrination by the other parent (almost exclusively as part of a child custody dispute) and the child's own attempts to denigrate the target parent.[1] Gardner introduced the term in a 1985 paper, describing a cluster of symptoms he had observed during the early 1980s.[1]

Parental alienation syndrome has the support of groups of parents who have been separated from their children by the law, some defending lawyers handling cases of divorce and some professionals who work in contested divorce cases holding that children are manipulated to make false allegations.

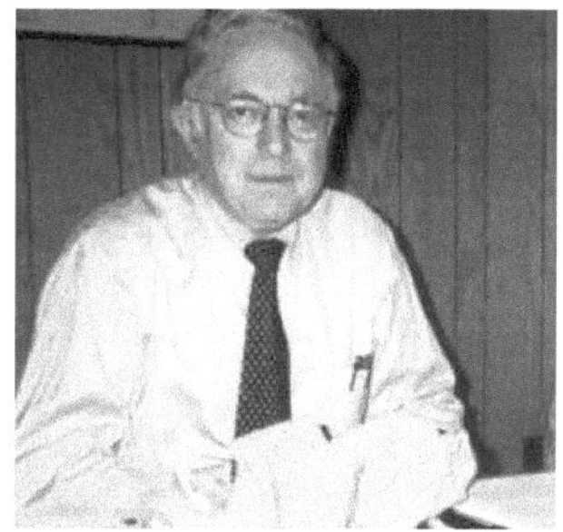

Richard A. Gardner coined the expression "parental alienation syndrome"

However, parental alienation syndrome is not recognized as a disorder by the medical or legal communities and Gardner's theory and related research have been extensively criticized by legal and mental health scholars for lacking scientific validity and reliability.[2] [3] [4] [5] [6] However, the separate but related concept of parental alienation, the estrangement of a child from a parent, is recognized as a dynamic in some divorcing families.[2] [7] [8]

The admissibility of PAS has been rejected by an expert review panel and the Court of Appeal of England and Wales in the United Kingdom and Canada's Department of Justice recommends against its use, but has appeared in some family court disputes in the United States.[9] [10] Gardner portrayed PAS as well accepted by the judiciary and having set a variety of precedents, but legal analysis of the actual cases indicates this claim was incorrect.[6]

No professional association has recognized PAS as a relevant medical syndrome or mental disorder, and it is not listed in the American Psychiatric Association's *Diagnostic and Statistical Manual of Mental Disorders* or the International Statistical Classification of Diseases and Related Health Problems of the WHO.

Initial description

Parental alienation syndrome was a term coined by child psychiatrist Richard A. Gardner drawing upon his clinical experiences since the early 1980s.[1] The concept of one parent attempting to separate their child from the other parent as punishment or part of a divorce have been described since at least the 1940s,[2] [8] but Gardner was the first to define a specific syndrome. In a 1985 article, he defined PAS as "...a disorder that arises primarily in the context of child-custody disputes. Its primary manifestation is the child's campaign of denigration against the parent, a campaign that has no justification. The disorder results from the combination of indoctrinations by the alienating parent and the child's own contributions to the vilification of the alienated parent"[1] also stating that the indoctrination may be deliberate or unconscious on the part of the alienating parent.[11] [12] PAS was originally developed as an explanation for the increase in the number of reports of child abuse in the 1980s.[13] [14] Gardner initially believed that parents (usually mothers) made false accusations of child abuse and sexual abuse against the other parent (usually fathers) in order to prevent further contact between them.[15] [16] While Gardner initially described the mother was the alienator in 90% of PAS cases, he later stated both parents were equally likely to alienate.[13] [17] [18] He also later stated that in his experience accusations of sexual abuse were not present in the vast majority of cases of PAS.[14] The initial work was self-published by Gardner, but later papers were released in peer reviewed scientific journals.

Characteristics

Gardner described PAS as a preoccupation by the child with criticism and deprecation of a parent.[19] Gardner stated that PAS occurs when, in the context of child custody disputes, one parent deliberately or unconsciously attempts to alienate a child from the other parent.[20] According to Gardner, PAS is characterized by a cluster of eight symptoms that appear in the child. These include a campaign of denigration and hatred against the targeted parent; weak, absurd, or frivolous rationalizations for this deprecation and hatred; lack of the usual ambivalence about the targeted parent; strong assertions that the decision to reject the parent is theirs alone (the "independent-thinker phenomenon"); reflexive support of the favored parent in the conflict; lack of guilt over the treatment of the alienated parent; use of borrowed scenarios and phrases from the alienating parent; and the denigration not just of the targeted parent but also to that parent's extended family and friends.[12] [17] [21] Despite frequent citations of these factors in scientific literature, "the value ascribed to these factors has not been explored with professionals in the field."[22]

Gardner and others have divided PAS into mild, moderate and severe levels. The number and severity of the eight symptoms displayed increase through the different levels. The recommendations for management differ according to the severity level of the child's symptoms. While a diagnosis of PAS is made based on the child's symptoms, Gardner stated that any change in custody should be based primarily on the symptom level of the alienating parent.[23] In mild cases, there is some parental programming against the targeted parent, but little or no disruption of visitation, and Gardner did not recommend court-ordered visitation. In moderate cases, there is more parental programming and greater resistance to visits with the targeted parent. Gardner recommended that primary custody remain with the programming parent if the brainwashing was expected to be discontinued, but if not, that custody should be transferred to the targeted parent. In addition, therapy with the child to stop alienation and remediate the damaged relationship with the targeted parent was recommended. In severe cases, children display most or all of the 8 symptoms, and will refuse steadfastly to visit the targeted parent, including threatening to run away or commit suicide if the visitation is forced. Gardner recommended that the child be removed from the alienating parent's home into a transition home before moving into the home of the targeted parent. In addition, therapy for the child is recommended.[1] [21] [23] Gardner's proposed intervention for moderate and severe PAS, including court-ordered transfer to the alienated parent, fines, house arrest, incarceration, have been critiqued for their punitive nature towards the alienating parent and alienated child, and for the risk of abuse of power and violation of their civil rights.[24] [25] With time, Gardner revised his views and expressed less support for the most aggressive management strategies.[24]

Reception

Gardner's original formulation, which labeled mothers almost exclusively as the alienating parent, was endorsed by fathers' rights groups, as it allowed fathers to explain the reluctance of their children to visit them and assign blame to their former wives.[24] [26] In contrast, women's groups criticized the syndrome, concerned that it permitted abusers to claim that allegations of abuse by mother or child were reflective of brainwashing.[24] Gardner himself emphasized that PAS only applied in situations where there was no actual abuse or neglect had not occurred,[6] [27] but by 1998, noted an increase in the awareness of PAS had led to an increase in its misapplication as an exculpatory legal maneuver.[11]

PAS has been cited in high-conflict divorce and child custody cases, particularly as a defense against accusations of domestic violence or sexual abuse.[4] [21] The status of the syndrome, and thus its admissibility in the testimony of experts, has been the subject of dispute about the extent to which PAS has been accepted by the professionals in the field, as well as a scientific methodology that is testable, has been tested, has a known error rate, has been published and is peer-reviewed.[21]

PAS has not been accepted by experts in child advocacy or the study of child abuse[5] or legal scholars.[6] In psychology the reception is mixed. Many experts such as Richard Warshak argue for it. PAS has been extensively criticized by members of the legal and mental health community, who state that PAS should not be admissible in child custody hearings based on both science and law.[6] [4] [5] [21] [28]

PAS is not recognized by the American Medical Association or the American Psychiatric Association.[6] [14] [15] [29] The American Psychological Association declined to give a position on PAS, but raised concerns over its lack of supporting data and how the term is used[30] and the APA's 1996 Presidential Task Force on Violence and the Family expressed concern that custody evaluators use PAS as a means of giving custody to fathers despite a history of violence, a concern shared by other commentators.[4] [31] [32] The United States National Council of Juvenile and Family Court Judges rejected PAS, recommending it not be used for the consideration of child custody issues.[26]

Absence from the *DSM*

PAS is not included in the American Psychiatric Association's *Diagnostic and Statistical Manual of Mental Disorders* (DSM-IV).[6] [14] [15] [29] Gardner and others have lobbied for its inclusion in the next revision of the manual.[17] [33] In 2001, Gardner argued that when the DSM-IV was released there was insufficient research to include PAS, but since then there have been enough scientific articles and attention to PAS that it merited being taken seriously.[17] A survey of American custody evaluators published in 2007 found that half of the respondents disagreed with its inclusion, while a third thought it should be.[12] A related formulation, parental alienation disorder, has been proposed as well; it was suggested that inclusion of PAS in the DSM-5 would promote research and appropriate treatment, as well as reduce misuse of a valid and reliable construct.[2] When a draft version of the DSM-5 was released in 2010, PAS was not included,[33] though parental alienation disorder does appear as a "Condition Proposed by Outside Sources" to be reviewed by a working group.[34]

Scientific status

Gardner's formulation of PAS is critiqued as lacking a scientific basis,[35] [36] [37] and as a hypothesis whose proponents have failed to meet the scientific burden of proof to merit acceptance.[6] [35] [37] The first publications about PAS were self-published and not peer reviewed,[8] and though subsequent articles have been published in peer reviewed journals, most have consisted of anecdotal evidence in the form of case studies;[38] [39] in addition, the limited research into PAS has lacked evidence of its validity and reliability.[4] [5] The lack of objective research and replication, falsifiability, and independent publication has led to claims that PAS is pseudoscience or junk science.[3] [35] [36] Proponents of PAS concur that large scale systematic controlled studies into PAS's validity and reliability are required,[8] [12] [40] supplementing a single small study in 2004 which suggested practitioners could come to a consensus based on written reports.[28]

The theoretical foundation of PAS has been described as incomplete, simplistic and erroneous for ignoring the multiple factors (including the behaviors of the child, parents and other family members) that may contribute to parental alienation, family dysfunction and a breakdown in attachment between a parent and a child.[8] [13] [31] [38] [41] In this view, PAS confuses a child's developmental reaction to a divorce with psychosis, vastly overstates the number of false allegations of child sexual abuse, ignores the scientific literature suggesting most allegations of child sexual abuse are well founded and thus well-meaning efforts to protect a child from an abusive parent, exaggerates the damaging effects of parental alienation on children and proposes an unsupported and endangering remedy for PAS.[4] [28] Concern has been expressed that PAS lacks adequate scientific support to be considered a syndrome and that Gardner has promoted PAS as a syndrome based on a vague clustering of behaviors.[8] [15] Despite concerns about the validity of testimony regarding PAS, it has been inappropriately viewed as reliable by family court judges.[6] Proponents of PAS and others agree that using the designation of syndrome may be inappropriate as it implies more scientific legitimacy than it currently deserves.[19] [24] [40]

While PAS is not accepted as a syndrome, parental alienation is a somewhat less controversial dynamic that has also appeared in the mental health and legal literature.[22] [24] Since Gardner proposed PAS, other researchers in the field have suggested focusing less on diagnosing a syndrome and more on what has been described as the "alienated child," and the dynamics of the situation that have contributed to the alienation.[13] [24]

Clinical status

PAS has been criticized for making clinical work with children who are alienated more confusing[8] and Gardner's analysis has been criticized for inappropriately assigning all responsibility of the child's behavior to one parent when the child's behavior is oftentimes, but not always, the result of a dynamic in which both parents and the child play a role.[25] [41]

Gardner disagreed with criticism of PAS as overly simplistic, stating that while there are a wide variety of causes on why a child may become alienated from a parent, the primary etiological factor in cases of PAS is the brainwashing parent, and that otherwise, there is no PAS.[11] Gardner also stated that those initially critical of PAS for being a caricature were not directly involved with families in custody disputes and that criticisms of this nature faded by the late 1980s because the disorder was widespread.[1]

Gender

PAS has been criticized by for being sexist, being used by fathers to marginalize legitimate fears and concerns about abuse, and women's groups and others oppose the legitimacy of PAS as a danger to children.[31] After his initial publications, Gardner revised his theory to make fathers and mothers equally likely to alienate or be indoctrinators and disagreed that recognition of PAS is sexist. Gardner later indicated he believed men were equally likely to be PAS indoctrinators.[11] Studies of children and adults labelled as suffering from PAS have suggested that mothers were more likely than fathers to be the alienator.[12]

In courts

Brazil is the only country whose laws recognize and condemns the SAP.[42]

Canada

Early Canadian court cases accepted expert opinions about PAS, used the term "syndrome" and concurred with Gardner's theory that only one parent was fully responsible for it. Gardner testified in one case (Fortin v. Major, 1996) but the court did not accept his opinion, concluding that the child was not alienated based on the evaluation of a court-appointed expert who, unlike Gardner, had met with the family members.[24] More recent cases, while accepting the concept of alienation, have noted the lack of recognition in the DSM-IV, and have generally avoided "syndrome" terminology, emphasizing that changes in custody are stressful for the child and should only occur in the most severe cases.[24] A 2006 research report by the Canadian Department of Justice described PAS as "empirically unsupported" and favored a different framework for dealing with issues of alienation that has more research support.[43] Decisions about possible parental alienation are considered a legal decision, to be determined by the judge based on the facts of the case, rather than a diagnosis made by a mental health professional. There is recognition that rejection of a parent is a complex issue, and that a distinction must be made between pathological alienation and reasonable estrangement.[24]

United Kingdom

In the United Kingdom, the admissibility concerning the evaluation of PAS was rejected both in an expert review,[44] and by the Court of Appeal.[9] [10]

United States

PAS has been cited as part of the child custody determination process in the United States.[9] Based on the evaluation of PAS, courts in the US have awarded sole custody to some fathers.[6] PAS has been challenged under the Frye test, to evaluate if it has been accepted by the scientific community.[6] [45] Despite Gardner claiming PAS was generally accepted by the scholarly community and passed the Frye test in two states,[11] a 2006 analysis of court cases involving PAS and cited by Gardner concluded that these decisions did not set legal precedent, that PAS is viewed negatively in most legal scholarship, and that Gardner's writings do not support the existence of PAS. Of sixty-four precedent-bearing cases, only two decisions, both in New York State and both in criminal courts actually set precedents. Both held PAS inadmissible and one case found that PAS failed the Frye test as the appropriate professional community did not generally accept; this decision was upheld in an appellate court. Gardner listed fifty cases on his website that he claimed set precedents that made PAS admissible, but none actually did; forty-six set no precedents or did not discuss admissibility and the remaining four were problematic. One case stated that PAS passed the Frye test, but the appeal did not discuss the Frye test and actually "[threw] out the words 'parental alienation syndrome'" and focused on the "willingness and ability of each parent to facilitate and encourage a close and continuing relationship between the parents and the child". In the second case, the appellate court did not discuss PAS; the third case specifically chose not to discuss the admissibility of PAS and the fourth made no decision on PAS.[6]

References

[1] Gardner, RA (2001). "Parental Alienation Syndrome (PAS): Sixteen Years Later" (http://www.fact.on.ca/Info/pas/gard01b.htm). *Academy Forum* **45** (1): 10–12. . Retrieved 2009-03-31.

[2] Bernet, W (2008). "Parental Alienation Disorder and DSM-V". *The American Journal of Family Therapy* **36** (5): 349–366. doi:10.1080/01926180802405513.

[3] Faller, KC (1998). "The parental alienation syndrome: What is it and what data support it?" (http://www.leadershipcouncil.org/docs/Faller1998.pdf) (pdf). *Child Maltreatment* **3** (2): 100–115. doi:10.1177/1077559598003002005. .

[4] Bruch, CS (2001). "Parental Alienation Syndrome and Parental Alienation: Getting It Wrong in Child Custody Cases" (http://www.law.ucdavis.edu/faculty/Bruch/files/fam353_06_Bruch_527_552.pdf) (pdf). *Family Law Quarterly* **35** (527): 527–552. .

[5] Wood, CL (1994). "The parental alienation syndrome: a dangerous aura of reliability" (http://fact.on.ca/Info/pas/wood94.htm). *Loyola of Los Angeles Law Review* **29**: 1367–1415. . Retrieved 2008-04-12.

[6] Hoult, JA (2006). "The Evidentiary Admissibility of Parental Alienation Syndrome: Science, Law, and Policy" (http://papers.ssrn.com/sol3/papers.cfm?abstract_id=910267). *Children's Legal Rights Journal* **26** (1). .

[7] Rohrbaugh, Joanna Bunker (2008). *A comprehensive guide to child custody evaluations: mental health and legal perspectives*. Berlin: Springer. pp. 399–438 (http://books.google.com/books?id=0W3QEqFWXdYC&pg=PA399). ISBN 0-387-71893-1.

[8] Warshak, RA (2001). "Current controversies regarding parental alienation syndrome" (http://www.rhfinc.org.au/docs/controversies.pdf) (pdf). *American Journal of Forensic Psychology* **19** (3): 29–59. .

[9] Fortin, Jane (2003). *Children's Rights and the Developing Law*. Cambridge University Press. pp. 263 (http://books.google.ca/books?id=etLxpQQQgocC&pg=PA263). ISBN 9780521606486.

[10] Bainham, Andrew (2005). *Children: The Modern Law*. Jordans. pp. 161 (http://books.google.ca/books?id=FIFWXhTi5AYC&pg=PA161). ISBN 9780853089391.

[11] Gardner, Richard (2004). "Commentary on Kelly and Johnston's The Alienated Child: A Reformulation of Parental Alienation Syndrome" (http://coleur.googlepages.com/GardnerrRichardACommentaryonKellyand.pdf) (pdf). *Family Court Review* **42** (4): 611–21. doi:10.1177/1531244504268711. .

[12] Baker, AJL (2007). "Knowledge and Attitudes About the Parental Alienation Syndrome: A Survey of Custody Evaluators". *American Journal of Family Therapy* **35** (1): 1–19. doi:10.1080/01926180600698368.

[13] Jaffe, PG; Lemon NKD; Poisson SE (2002). *Child Custody & Domestic Violence*. SAGE Publications. pp. 52–54 (http://books.google.ca/books?id=bbZmp7ALOq4C&pg=PA52). ISBN 9780761918264.

[14] Dallam, SJ (1999). "The Parental Alienation Syndrome: Is It Scientific?" (http://www.leadershipcouncil.org/1/res/dallam/3.html). In St. Charles E; Crook L. *Expose: The failure of family courts to protect children from abuse in custody disputes*. Our Children Our Children Charitable Foundation. .

[15] Caplan, PJ (2004). "What is it that's being called Parental Alienation Syndrome". In Caplan PJ; Cosgrove L. *Bias in psychiatric diagnosis*. Rowman & Littlefield. pp. 62 (http://books.google.ca/books?id=6XPLguPHzHoC&pg=PA62). ISBN 9780765700018.

[16] Brown, T; Renata A (2007). *Child Abuse and Family Law: Understanding the Issues Facing Human Service and Legal Professionals*. Allen & Unwin. pp. 11–12 (http://books.google.ca/books?id=USkixwfefC0C&pg=PA11). ISBN 9781865087313.

[17] Gardner, RA (2002). "Denial of the Parental Alienation Syndrome Also Harms Women". *American Journal of Family Therapy* **30** (3): 191–202. doi:10.1080/019261802753577520.

[18] Baker AJL (2007). *Adult children of parental alienation syndrome: breaking the ties that bind*. New York: W. W. Norton & Company. ISBN 0-393-70519-6.

[19] Ackerman, Ph.D, Marc J. (2002). *Clinician's Guide to Child Custody Evaluations* (http://books.google.com/?id=q9E_rg94Cs4C&pg=PA73). John Wiley and Sons,. pp. 73–82. ISBN 9780471150916. .

[20] Jaffe, Peter G.; Lemon, Nancy K. D., Poisson, Samantha E. (2002). *Child Custody & Domestic Violence* (http://books.google.com/?id=bbZmp7ALOq4C&pg=PA52). SAGE Publications. pp. 52–54. ISBN 9780761918264. .

[21] Walker, LEA; Brantley KL; Rigsbee JA (2004). "A Critical Analysis of Parental Alienation Syndrome and Its Admissibility in the Family Court". *Journal of Child Custody* **1** (2): 47–74. doi:10.1300/J190v01n02_03.

[22] Bow, JN; Gould JW; Flens JR (2009). "Examining Parental Alienation in Child Custody Cases: A Survey of Mental Health and Legal Professionals". *The American Journal of Family Therapy* **37** (2): 127–145. doi:10.1080/01926180801960658.

[23] Gardner, Richard A. (2006). "Introduction". In Gardner, Richard A.; Sauber, S. Richard; Lorandos, Demosthenes. *The International Handbook of Parental Alienation Syndrome: Conceptual, Clinical And Legal Considerations*. Charles C. Thomas. pp. 5–11. ISBN 978-0398076474.

[24] Bala, Nicholas; Fidler, Barbara-Jo; Goldberg, Dan; Houston, Claire (2007). "Alienated Children and Parental Separation: Legal Responses in Canada's Family Courts" (http://scholar.google.ca/scholar?hl=en&lr=&q=info:pwdqOnkrT8IJ:scholar.google.com/&output=viewport&pg=1). *Queen's Law Journal* **38**: 79–138. .

[25] Johnston, JR; Kelly JB (2004). "Rejoinder to Gardner's Commentary on Kelly and Johnston's 'The Alienated Child: A Reformulation of Parental Alienation Syndrome'" (http://www3.interscience.wiley.com/journal/118817173/abstract?CRETRY=1&SRETRY=0). *Family Court Review* **42** (4): 622–628. doi:10.1111/j.174-1617.2004.tb01328.x. .

[26] Ottaman, A; Lee R (2008). "Fathers' rights movement". In Edleson JL; Renzetti, CM. *Encyclopedia of Interpersonal Violence*. SAGE Publications. pp. 252 (http://books.google.ca/books?id=BOKAMXEA_jQC&pg=PA252). ISBN 978-1412918008.

[27] Gardner, RA (1998). "Recommendations for Dealing with Parents who Induce a Parental Alienation Syndrome in their Children". *Journal of Divorce & Remarriage* **28** (3/4): 1–21. doi:10.1300/J087v28n03_01.

[28] Drozd, L (2009). "Rejection in cases of abuse or alienation in divorcing families". In Galatzer-Levy RM; Kraus L & Galatzer-Levy J. *The Scientific Basis of Child Custody Decisions, 2nd Edition*. John Wiley & Sons. pp. 403–416 (http://books.google.ca/books?id=_-z0OIjyPyEC&pg=PA403). ISBN 9780470038581.

[29] Comeford, L (2009). "Fatherhood Movements". In O'Brien J. *Encyclopedia of Gender and Society*. **1**. SAGE Publications. pp. 285 (http://books.google.ca/books?id=_nyHS4WyUKEC&pg=PA285). ISBN 9781412909167.

[30] "APA Statement on Parental Alienation Syndrome" (http://www.apa.org/news/press/releases/2008/01/pas-syndrome.aspx). Washington, DC: American Psychological Association. 1996. . Retrieved 2009-03-31.

[31] Sparta, SN; Koocher GP (2006). *Forensic Mental Health Assessment of Children and Adolescents*. Oxford University Press. pp. 83 (http://books.google.ca/books?id=6bmBtQ2Zl-IC&pg=PA83), 219–221 (http://books.google.ca/books?id=6bmBtQ2Zl-IC&pg=PA219). ISBN 9780195145847.

[32] "American Psychological Association Presidential Task Force on Violence And The Family" (http://web.archive.org/web/20000307233013/www.apa.org/pi/pii/familyvio/issue5.html). American Psychological Association. 1996. Archived from the original (http://www.apa.org/pi/pii/familyvio/issue5.html) on 2000-03-07. .

[33] Rotstein, Gary (February 15, 2010). "Mental health professionals getting update on definitions" (http://www.post-gazette.com/pg/10046/1036018-114.stm). *Pittsburgh Post-Gazette*. . Retrieved 2 March 2010.

[34] "Conditions Proposed by Outside Sources" (http://www.dsm5.org/ProposedRevisions/Pages/ConditionsProposedbyOutsideSources.aspx). American Psychiatric Association. 2010. . Retrieved 2010-03-20.

[35] Emery, RE (2005). "Parental Alienation Syndrome: Proponents bear the burden of proof" (http://www.ncdsv.org/images/PASProponentsBeartheBurdenofProof_Emery_2005.pdf) (pdf). *Family Court Review* **43** (1): 8–13. .

[36] Bond, Richard (2008). *The Lingering Debate Over the Parental Alienation Syndrome Phenomenon*. **4**. Journal of Child Custody. pp. 37–54.

[37] Martindale, David; Gould, Jonathan W. (2007). *The Art and Science of Child Custody Evaluations*. New York: The Guilford Press. ISBN 1-59385-488-9.

[38] Ackerman MJ (2001). *Clinician's guide to child custody evaluations*. New York: John Wiley & Sons. pp. 73–82 (http://books.google.ca/ books?id=q9E_rg94Cs4C&pg=PA73). ISBN 0-471-39260-X.

[39] Ragland, ER; Fields H (2003). "Parental Alienation Syndrome: What Professionals Need to Know Part 1 of 2 Update" (http://www.ndaa. org/publications/newsletters/update_volume_16_number_6_2003.html). *American Prosecutors Research Institute Newsletter* **16** (6). .

[40] Warshak, Richard A.. "Bringing sense to Parental Alienation: A Look at the Disputes and the Evidence". *Family Law Quarterly* **37** (2): 273–301.

[41] Waldron, KH; Joanis DE (1996). "Understanding and Collaboratively Treating Parental Alienation Syndrome" (http://fact.on.ca/Info/ pas/waldron.htm). *American Journal of Family Law* **10**: 121–133. .

[42] *A nova lei da alienação parental* (http://psicologiajuridica.org/archives/730). Psicología jurídica y forense. 2010. . Retrieved 2011-05-05.

[43] Jaffe, PG; Crooks CV & Bala N (2006) (pdf). *Making Appropriate Parenting Arrangements in Family Violence Cases: Applying the Literature to Identify Promising Practices* (http://www.justice.gc.ca/eng/pi/pad-rpad/rep-rap/2005_3/2005_3.pdf). Department of Justice. . Retrieved 2009-05-05.

[44] Sturge, C; Glaser D (2000). "Contact and domestic violence – the experts' court report". *Family Law* **615**.

[45] Myers, John E. B. (2005). *Myers on evidence in child, domestic, and elder abuse cases*. Gaithersburg, Md: Aspen Publishers. pp. 415 (http:/ /books.google.com/books?id=-krZZF9dl-sC&pg=PA415). ISBN 0-7355-5668-7.

External links

- Parental alienation syndrome (http://www.dmoz.org//Society/People/Men/Issues/Fathers'_Rights/ Divorce_and_Custody/Parental_Alienation_Syndrome//) at the Open Directory Project

Family_law

Family law is an area of the law that deals with family-related issues and domestic relations including:

- the nature of marriage, civil unions, and domestic partnerships;
- issues arising throughout marriage, including spousal abuse, legitimacy, adoption, surrogacy, child abuse, and child abduction
- the termination of the relationship and ancillary matters including divorce, annulment, property settlements, alimony, and parental responsibility orders (in the United States, child custody and visitation, child support and alimony awards).
- Paternity fraud and testing
- Juvenile adjudication

This list is by no means dispositive of the potential issues that come through the family court system. In many jurisdictions in the United States, the family courts see the most crowded dockets. Litigants representative of all social and economic classes are parties within the system.

For the conflict of laws elements dealing with transnational and interstate issues, see marriage (conflict), divorce (conflict) and nullity (conflict).

See also

- Alimony
- Paternity fraud
- Merger doctrine (family law)
- supervised visitation

Specific jurisdictions

- Algerian Family Code
- Family Court of Australia

  - Australian family law
- Family Law Act (Alberta, Canada)
- Family law system in England and Wales

  - The Children Act 1989
  - Sir Morris Finer - Report on One Parent Families
- Malian Family Code
- Mudawana (The Moroccan Family Code).
- Civil Code of the Philippines

Further reading

- Testimony of Barbara DaFoe Whitehead, Ph.D, Co-Director, National Marriage Project Rutgers University, before US Senate Subcommitee [1]
- Wallerstein, Judith, Ph.D., "The Unexpected Legacy of Divorce", an analysis of the long-term effect of divorce on children; NPR interview (2000) [2]

References

[1] http://marriage.rutgers.edu/Publications/Pub%20Whitehead%20Testimony%20Apr%2004.htm

[2] http://www.pbs.org/newshour/conversation/july-dec00/wallerstein_12-19.htm

Article Sources and Contributors

Parents'_rights_movement *Source*: http://en.wikipedia.org/w/index.php?title=Parents%27_rights_movement *Contributors*: Dr.enh, Freechild, Michael H 34, Miq, Peculiar Light, Philosopher, Sardanaphalus, 1 anonymous edits

Civil_rights_movement *Source*: http://en.wikipedia.org/w/index.php?title=Civil_rights_movement *Contributors*: --, April, 21655, 28421u2232nfenfcenc, Abce2, Aberdonian99, Abune, Addshore, Aeusoes1, Ahoerstemeier, Aitias, Aktron, Alansohn, Aleenf1, Alex.muller, Alfio, Alice.haugen, Amadscientist, Amire80, Amorymeltzer, Ancheta Wis, Andonic, Andrewpmk, Animum, Anoderate1, AnonGuy, Anonymous Dissident, Antandrus, Antonio Lopez, Apardee, Arakunem, Arctic Night, Arre, Art LaPella, Artaddict93, Asdfj, Astanto, Aurick, AvicAWB, Avono, Avs5221, BaronGrackle, BarretB, Barticus88, Beaumont, Beland, Bencherlite, Bender235, Beyourbest, Bhadani, Bickytoria, Bility, Biruitorul, Blair Bonnett, Blobecek, Blobglob, Bluedenim, Bobfrombrockley, Bobo192, Bodnotbod, Boing! said Zebedee, Bongwarrior, Boothy443, BrianKnez, Brianga, Brit hideaway, BryanFrazar, Bsadowski1, Bubba73, Bukubku, CWY2190, Calesyndrome, Caltas, Calvin 1998, Camille Harrigan, Can't sleep, clown will eat me, Canadian-Bacon, CanadianLinuxUser, Canterbury Tail, CapitalSasha, Capricorn42, Catgut, Cbustapeck, Ccson, Cgingold, ChemGardener, Chickyfuzz14, Chris'sgirl2006, ClydeOnline, Coffee, Colonies Chris, Cometstyles, Cool Blue, Crazy Boris with a red beard, Cst17, Cunningham, DMacks, Daniel 1992, Dargen, Davewild, DavidPaulHamilton, Deeceevoice, Delirium, DemitreusFrontwest, Dgies, Difluoroethene, Dinnertimeok, Dipto.M, Discospinster, DocWatson42, Doulos Christos, Dreadstar, Drooling Sheep, Dustingc, Dv82matt, E.G., EVula, Ecelan, Edivorce, EdoDodo, Edunoramus, Edward321, Eeekster, Eh kia, Ejosse1, El C, Epbr123, Eurytus, Everyking, Extransit, Extraordinary, Fairlane75, Faradayplank, Fightindaman, Flyguy649, Fods12, Foxj, Fram, FrancoGG, Fraser1390, Fratrep, Fusionmix, GT5162, Gaidheal, Gail, Gaius Cornelius, Gakusha, Germanforces123456789, Gfxguy, Giants27, Gilliam, Ginsengbomb, Glaze012, Gmaxwell, Gobonobo, Green meklar, Grimey109, Groovydude777, Gtstricky, Guoguo12, Gurch, Gurchzilla, HAMM, Hadal, Hadrianheugh, Haemo, Helenalex, Hersfold, Hobartimus, Hotmonkey25, Hut 8.5, IRP, Icairns, Imcool596, Imran, Indefatigable, IndulgentReader, Ixfd64, J Martin81, J.delanoy, JForget, JHunterJ, JaGa, Jacklee, Jasonyoon5251, JayJasper, Jayjayjaycrashjay, Jeepday, Jemather, Jerzy, Jessie baby 13, Jfknrh, JimVC3, Jipajappa, Joe Decker, John Quiggin, John254, Jujumagumbo, Jujutacular, Juliancolton, Justincannon4, KPH2293, Kazayta, Keilana, Keithgreer, Kesac, Kevin j, Khalidkhoso, Kikodawgzz, Kikodawgzzz, King of Hearts, Kingpin13, KnowledgeOfSelf, Kubigula, Kukini, Kuru, La Pianista, Landon1980, Laqualla, Lea Orr, LeaveSleaves, Lectonar, LedgendGamer, Leif, Lemniwinks, Levangel, LibLord, Lightmouse, Lights, Linnell, Little Mountain 5, Littlelass1414, Littlesana, Longhair, Lopakhin, Lquilter, Lucid dre4m, LuigiManiac, Luna Santin, MER-C, Marcan, Marcheseis, Marek69, Marionlad, Mark Arsten, Markgage, Mboverload, Mentifisto, Merope, Metre01, Midgrid, Mike123090, Milesli, Mimzy1990, Moderate2008, Monkeyblue, Montanean, MrFish, Mrceleb2007, MsDivagin, Mspraveen, Munoz101, Musiqueue, NHJG, Nburden, NewEnglandYankee, Nixeagle, Nlu, Noah Salzman, Ntennis, Nv8200p, OhSoOrdinary, Omicronpersei8, One Night In Hackney, Osprey39, Otisjimmy1, Oxymoron83, PCock, Padraig, Paine, Paranomia, Parkwells, Party, Past Outcast, Pat878, PaulGarner, Pb30, Persian Poet Gal, Pfhorrest, Philip Trueman, PiMaster3, Podpet24, PonchoVineta, Prashanthns, Prolog, Purpleslog, Quindie, Qwertypoiuyman, Qxz, R'n'B, Racepacket, Radon210, RandomP, RandomXYZb, Randy Kryn, Razorflame, Rcduggan, Recognizance, Red King, Reeseseatsbabies, RexNL, Riana, Rich Farmbrough, Rigadoun, Rjensen, Rjwilmsi, Rl, RodC, Rokfaith, Ronhjones, Rosemaryamey, Rrburke, SGGH, ST47, Saalstin, SamEV, Samsara, Sandstein, Satori Son, Scartol, SchfiftyThree, SchnitzelMannGreek, Sciurinæ, Semperf, Senator Palpatine, Seraphimblade, Setanta747, Setanta747 (locked), Shenme, Shinpah1, Shoemaker's Holiday, Silly rabbit, Simesa, Sionus, Sir Vicious, SkerHawx, Sketchmoose, Skixz, Slon02, Sluzzelin, Smalljim, SmartGuy Old, Snigbrook, Snowolf, SoLando, Soetermans, Somearemoreequal, Soxwon, Staffwaterboy, Stephenb, Steven Zhang, Stoopkitty, Tanthalas39, Tayg0, Tempodivalse, That Guy, From That Show!, The Anome, The Cunctator, The PIPE, The Rambling Man, The Thing That Should Not Be, The sock that should not be, TheRaven7, Theda, Theoldanarchist, Thingg, Thop100, Tiddly Tom, Tide rolls, Tom Radulovich, Tom harrison, TonyTheTiger, Tozoku, Trevor MacInnis, Tristan123456789, Truk425, TutterMouse, Ugur Basak, Ukexpat, Ulric1313, Valenciano, Vanished 6551232, Venu62, Viriditas, WadeSimMiser, Waggers, Watersoftheoasis, Wavelength, Welsh, Wikicaz, Wikipediatastic, Willm666, Wimt, Woohookitty, Wtmitchell, Xtmnxzombiex, Yahel Guhan, Yamamoto Ichiro, Yboord028, Yintan, Zapvet, Zereshk, ZimZalaBim, Ziusudra, Zzuuzz, 1238 anonymous edits

Child_custody *Source*: http://en.wikipedia.org/w/index.php?title=Child_custody *Contributors*: 7&6=thirteen, A. B., Analcka, Andy king50, Another n00b, Antixt, Ariwara, BMF81, Bigrob31620, BozMo, Briman1, Burrburr, COMPFUNK2, Calabe1992, Casey Abell, Cervantescid, Christobalclemente, Connect.Media, Correogsk, CustodieMinori, Cybermud, DanielCragun, David91, Dchesley, Deadspirit90, Dk1965, DrParkash, Dwj119, EdBever, Eeekster, Elizmartin, Enriquem111, Epeefleche, Escape Orbit, Esprit Segue, FRContributor, Finn Bjørklid, Frehley, Funnyguy1021, Goldenrowley, Golf Bravo, Hu12, Intern0323, Israelbeach, JJames82, Jimtaip, Jonkerz, Justice12, KGasso, Kgw2, Kittybrewster, L.tak, LM03, Ladler, Leventio, Lotje, Martrn, Mer nv, Michael H 34, Mike6271, MikeRogers, Monkeyman, MrOllie, MrWhich, Newman Luke, Nick Number, Ohnoitsjamie, Parenttimenet, Paul foord, Pi.C.Noizecehx, Poisonotter, Poopdeck90210, Qst, Rabbie Barns, Red Denim, SAC, SamiKaero, Samuel Blanning, Sarah Dillon, Sardanaphalus, Searsmall, Slp1, StaticGull, Steven P Kemp, Stomache1, Tassedethe, The Hippie, Trantsbugle, USA02, Viking soul, Woohookitty, XavierBrieze, Yaelim, 92 anonymous edits

Best_interests *Source*: http://en.wikipedia.org/w/index.php?title=Best_interests *Contributors*: A. B., Achildsbestinterest, Agwiii, Alex756, Andycjp, BD2412, Catalytic111, Chris the speller, Chrisminter, Custodyiq, Cybermud, David91, Dekisugi, Eranb, Freechild, Granmom, Hephaestos, Jeffz, Joep Zander, Kevin Gorman, Kutera Genesis, LM03, Light current, Luvtheheaven, MacsBug, Markruffolo, Matthew Stannard, Miagirljmw14, Michael H 34, Mrbandrews, Neutrality, Niteowlneils, Ohnoitsjamie, PullUpYourSocks, Red Denim, Rhrad, SAC, Sam Hocevar, SamWigley, Sidhekin, Tabletop, Tooru, Trantsbugle, 33 anonymous edits

Mind_control *Source*: http://en.wikipedia.org/w/index.php?title=Mind_control *Contributors*: 168..., 37 cent, AGToth, AI, AManWithNoPlan, Aaron Kauppi, Abdul747, AbsolutDan, AdSR, Aenar, Aeternus, Aff123a, Alberto89m, Aldie, Altenmann, Anacapa, Anarchia, Andries, Andycjp, Anetode, Angie Y., Animeanonymous, Antaeus Feldspar, Anthere, AnthonyQBachler, AntiACM, Antidermis2319, Artful Dodger, Arthur Rubin, Arturo57, Aviatorpilotman, AvicAWB, Ayecee, B4Ctom1, BD2412, BabyDweezil, Babykk666, Badagnani, Beggining99998, Beland, Benlisquare, Bento00, Bert56, Bfinn, Bhuston, Bibliosophe, BigFatBuddha, Bilby, Blackvault, Blah999888, Blaswell, Bmclaughlin9, Bobblewik, Boodlesthecat, BozMo, BrightBlackHeaven, Btilm, Bubbha, Butros, Bytwerk, C.Fred, C14ism, CBDunkerson, CLW, Camillus McElhinney, CanadianCaesar, Casito, Cattus, Chaaalieboy, Chris Gair, Christian75, Cirt, Cmdrjameson, Cogpsych, Conversion script, Courcelles, CowboyDon, Cretog8, Crockspot, CronoDAS, Crosbiesmith, Crzrussian, Curps, Cybercobra, Cyrilglass, DANK (usurped), Damion, Danelo, Daniel J. Leivick, Dave souza, David91, Davodd, Dawnseeker2000, De728631, Denisarona, Dept of Alchemy, Descendall, DocWatson42, Dorian321, Dr01234, Drmies, EBlack, Earle Martin, Ed Poor, Edgar181, Eep², El C, ElijahBosley, Elmmapleoakpine, Eloquence, EmmDee, Eshaler, Eudj, ExitControl, ExtraBold, Eyu100, Fahrenheit451, Faramarz, Farry, Farstriker, Faust2007, Fefenous X, Feitclub, FeloniousMonk, Fences and windows, Fixentries, Flecko, Folajimi, Fortdj33, Fossa, Francesco Pozzi, Fredburks, FreeSilver, Froid, Funeral, Furrykef, GKurdina, Gaius Cornelius, GangofOne, Gary D, Gazpacho, Geni, Getheren, GossamerBliss, Grafen, GrandMattster, Green meklar, Greennature2, Greenrd, Gregbard, GregorB, Gtrmp, Guestpass, Guoguo12, Gwalla, HGB, Haley2841, Harburg, Heron, Hkhenson, I42, IdeArchos, Igoldste, Iiible, Imran, InShaneee, Inks.LWC, Irmgard, IsaacJ, JALockhart, JHFTC, JLMadrigal, JR Richard, JacquesPaul, Jambalaya, James Crippen, JamesBWatson, Janessae, Jarich, Jayen466, Jeremygbyrne, Jeremystalked, Jfdwolff, Jfurr1981, Jim101, JimmyT, Jiy, JmSchanck, Jmlthr, Jnk, JoeSmack, Johanneum, JohnGabriel1, Johnkarp, Johnuniq, Joie de Vivre, Jojhutton, Jonathan de Boyne Pollard, Jossi, Jrtayloriv, Juan c vallejos, Just Another Dan, Justanother, Kaisei, Kalexander, Karl gregory jones, KarlHeg, Kasreyn, Kchishol1970, Ketiltrout, Ketorin, Kevin, Khukri, Kidlittle, Kilva, Kingboyk, Kitfoxxe, Kittybrewster, Knowledge558, Knverma, Koavf, Kozuch, Kubigula, Kungfuadam, Lakefall, Laocoont, Larry_Sanger, Lattf, Lcarscad, Lemmey, Lensman1, Liberatus, Lightmouse, Llort, Looie496, Lowellian, Lupin, MER-C, Mabuse, Magister Mathematicae, Male1979, Mark Arsten, Maroux, Marskell, MartinHarper, Master Jay, Matthew, Mattisse, Maureen D, Maziotis, McGeddon, McSly, Mcra, Meco, MegX, Melaen, MercyBreeze, Mfigroid, Michael Hardy, Michaelpb, Middleman 77, Midgley, Mikeo, Mild Bill Hiccup, Missionable, Mmmmtmmmm, Modemac, Mr Christopher, Mr.Grave, MuZemike, MysteryDog, N3wt3stam3nt88, Nasnema, Ne0Freedom, Nehrams2020, Neilbeach, Nemonoman, Nerd42, Neski, Nezrok Braughler, Nightbit, Noformation, Nono64, NoychoH, Nuuon, Obyezyanka, Oliver Pereira, Olivier, Ombudsman, Onesius, Onorem, OpenToppedBus, Orenburg1, Ortolan88, Oskoch, PPdd, Paine Ellsworth, Pakaran, Pascal.Tesson, Patfitz, Patrick, Pcb21, Pedant17, Pegship, PelleSmith, Penbat, Per Olofsson, Perspective, Peter T.S., Peter Winnberg, Pgreenfinch, Pigman, Pion, Plagas, Pogosuicide, Popefauvexxiii, Populus, Premeditated Chaos, Prezbo, Q Valda, Qasrani, RandomRubikMan, Rebroad, Reconsider the static, RedWolf, Reddi, Redvers, RepublicanJacobite, ResearchEditor, ResidentAnthropologist, RexNL, Rich Farmbrough, Richard-of-Earth, Ricmarques, Rjanag, Rjwilmsi, Roadrunner, RobinEvans, Rursus, Rédacteur Tibet, S. M. Sullivan, Saganaki-, Sam Hocevar, Samkass, Sannse, Scarian, Schneelocke, Sciberking, Sebastian scha., Senis, Senthryl, Sheilrod, Simetrical, Simon12, SiobhanHansa, Skier Dude, Skyzy, Sleigh, Sloth monkey, Smartse, Smee, Smilingman, SnappingTurtle, Sodium, Somewhatdazed, Spazure, Spearhead, Spencer, SqueakBox, StanfordProgrammer, Stefanomione, Stephenchou0722, Steve Dufour, Stevertigo, Stifle, Suidafrikaan, Suppressedminds, Susvolans, Sweetandy, Syvanen, Tanaats, TastyPoutine, Teh roflmaoer, Teh tennisman, Tekmaster1, Testbed, Texture, The Anome, The Golden Circle, The JPS, The Person Who Is Strange, The Rambling Man, The Rationalist, The Thing That Should Not Be, TheFBH, TheLeopard, ThePhantom, Thernlund, ThunderdanJP, Tide rolls, TimBentley, Titansolaris, Tmmullin, Tom harrison, Tom the Goober, Tommy2010, Torchiest, Transferofpower, Trivial, Trut-h-urts man, Tsuchiya Hikaru, Tumacama, Tzuhou, UltimatePyro, Urielw, User2004, UtherSRG, Van helsing, Veinor, Vertig-oh, Vingummi, Visite fortuitement prolongée, Voldemort, Volker89, WLU, Wavelength, Wayne Slam, Weaponbb7, Weazzel2828, WegianWarrior, Wekn reven i susej eht, Wenli, Werty892, Wiki alf, Wikiborg, Wikiguy1, WillOakland, Wilson2007, Wingover, Wiscados, Wizguru, Wizzerdd, Wmahan, Wn9mam, Woodrow Buzard, Woohookitty, WpZurp, XA-9, Xbvca, Xmmann, Y0u, Yono, Yotcmdr, Z205e501p, Zappaz, Zooplah, Zzuuzz, 700 anonymous edits

Massachusetts_Supreme_Judicial_Court *Source*: http://en.wikipedia.org/w/index.php?title=Massachusetts_Supreme_Judicial_Court *Contributors*: Acegikmo1, Assawyer, Axios023, Az29, BD2412, Bcorr, BigD527, Biruitorul, Bmclaughlin9, Briancua, Brianyoumans, CapitalR, CaribDigita, Chrism, Clb5880, Colonel Warden, CommonsDelinker, Dale Arnett, Domingo Portales, Drlowell, Dubhdara, Eastlaw, Emufarmers, FoekeNoppert, Fry1989, GabrielF, Gang14, Gblaz, GoldRingChip, Hirolovesswords, Hmains, Homagetocatalonia, Howcheng, Hydriotaphia, Ikip, Jessicapierce, JoeyBagODonuts, Jonathanrubin921, JustAGal, Lincolnite, M2545, Magicpiano, Muzi, Neutrality, P2Medic, Postdlf, Preslethe, R'n'B, RFD, Raj Fra, Rlquall, Rmhermen, Saaga, Sahasrahla, Sardanaphalus, Superm401, Svgalbertian, Swampyank, TJRC, Taco325i, Tassedethe, TonyTheTiger, Whitfield Larrabee, Wmcewenjr, Yellowdesk, 39 anonymous edits

Sabotage *Source*: http://en.wikipedia.org/w/index.php?title=Sabotage *Contributors*: 16@r, 1984, 98ui80i, AManWithNoPlan, Aaron Brenneman, Acerperi, AdjustShift, Alan ffm, Alexius08, AlphaPyro, Antandrus, Anthony Appleyard, Apeloverage, Art LaPella, Athaler, Atulsnischal, AwamerT, Beeblebrox, Bell031, Beta m, Bkell, Bluemoose, Bobsegii, BrianKnez, Bushytails, Butseriouslyfolks, CambridgeBayWeather, Careful With That Axe, Eugene, Carnildo, Chato, Chinasaur, Cjwright79, Cntras, Colonies Chris, Common Man, CommonsDelinker, Conversion script, Csl77, Cyan, Cyrius, DARTH SIDIOUS 2, DVdm, Dagnytaggartmoxie, Damian Yerrick, Danhussey, Dansuper, DetroitWobbly, Donreed, Drufin, Dysepsion, EchetusXe, EvelinaB,

Feddacheenee, Fhsssssss, Fieldday-sunday, Fixentries, Funandtrvl, FunnyMan3595, GCarty, Gob Lofa, Goffrie, Gogo Dodo, Grievre, Halibutt, HandsomeFella, Hank chapot, Heron, Hmains, Hvn0413, Ida Shaw, Ilikefood, Inter, Irishguy, Irpen, IshmaelMarcos, Ismaeeluk, JNW, JaGa, JamesBWatson, Janejellyroll, Jebba, John Price, Karada, Kirill Lokshin, KirinX, Knife Knut, Leonard G., Liftarn, Lightmouse, Lincolnite, Logologist, Long beach is in canadia, Lukepeterson, MC10, Malcolm Farmer, Martpol, Master Deusoma, Matthew, Matthewrbowker, Mayfly may fly, Maziotis, Mbc362, Melsaran, Memaster3, Mgaved, Michael Hardy, Mike Rosoft, Mike Schwartz, Mild Bill Hiccup, Mimihitam, Mission9801, Misza13, Monaarora84, Mrand, Muchness, Mufka, Mushed, Nabokov, NinjaKid, Nnh, Nobs01, OlEnglish, Onodevo, Otend, Paddingtonbaer, Pebbbles, Penbat, Philip Baird Shearer, Pit-yacker, RandomP, Reddi, Richard Myers, Richardson j, Rjwilmsi, Robsomebody, Ronhjones, Rossrs, SGBailey, Salahx, Salamurai, Salmanazar, Scientizzle, Sd31415, Sensemaker, Septagram, ShaunES, Skitzzo, Slysplace, Smb1001, Softlavender, Somercet, Spot87, Spywriter, Stefanomione, Stevertigo, Sum w0n, Suviljan, SvenGodo, The Merciful, Theda, ThinkBlue, Thismightbezach, Titsagreatday, Tommy2010, Umdenken, Varsil, Vianello, Vom, Wally, WarthogDemon, Wayland, Wiggy!, Woohookitty, Wred1str, Yaedaien, Yamaguchi, YanA, Youzwan, Zatoichi26, ZooFari, 225 anonymous edits

Parental_alienation_syndrome *Source*: http://en.wikipedia.org/w/index.php?title=Parental_alienation_syndrome *Contributors*: Aaron Kauppi, AdjustShift, Amcbride, Amorrow, Anacapa, Anaraug, Andycjp, Blanchardb, Bneidlinger, BozMo, Bzhb, Caiaffa, Cat Whisperer, Ckatz, Comazell, Cornell92, Darth Panda, Davecrosby uk, David91, Ddoomdoom, DeanTong, Dejudicibus, Desmay, Dinomite, Dreadstar, Durova, ERobson, Eastlaw, Endymionspilos, Epbr123, Ermeyers, Ervinn, Esprit Segue, Fainites, Faunas, GRuban, Gaius Cornelius, Gcr 2007, Georgius, Graham87, Hu12, Ilgiz, Imin2, ImperfectlyInformed, Informationonwomen, Ixfd64, JaGa, Jack-A-Roe, Jaluj, JaniceMT, JavierMC, Jenny Wong, Joep Zander, JohnClarknew, Jéské Couriano, Kintetsubuffalo, Kittybrewster, Lacatosias, LeoO3, Loneranger4justice, Lotterl, Lova Falk, Luis Dantas, MONGO, Magi2, Malick78, Markruffolo, Matthew Stannard, Melongrower, MercantorCoal, Mfreeny, Michael H 34, Mild Bill Hiccup, Mmpiking, Musical Linguist, Neutrality, Paul foord, Philosopher, Pilotguy, PinkCake, PrestonH, Rebel, Rebrane, ResearchEditor, Rich Farmbrough, Rjwilmsi, S-MorrisVP, SallyForth123, Search4Lancer, Searsmall, Sirrion, Slp1, Smith research, Someguy1221, Soultaco, SteveSims, Thu, Tito4000, Toswi82, Trish Wilson, Vannin, Vgy7ujm, WBoelter, WLU, West London Dweller, WhatamIdoing, William M. Connolley, Wissons, Wjohnsonva, Woohookitty, Wubrgamer, 161 anonymous edits

Family_law *Source*: http://en.wikipedia.org/w/index.php?title=Family_law *Contributors*: 5 Easy Pieces, A. B., Addw, Ahoerstemeier, Aj845, Alex.tan, Alex756, Amorrow, Ana1cka, Anonymouse99, Anyo Niminus, Apoc2400, Avjoska, BD2412, Bbatsell, Bearian, Beefalo, Beniamino, Berean Hunter, BigBen0, Blue-Haired Lawyer, Bonadea, Brianjones10, Caesura, Cameron Dewe, Caverslaw, CliffC, Cmdrjameson, Conversion script, Crackerjack, DJ Clayworth, Danger, David91, Debresser, DreamGuy, Dwj119, EdvensonConsulting, Efindel, El C, Epbr123, Erud, Familylaw99, FayssalF, FisherQueen, Fredbauder, Funandtrvl, G.Tenzing, GMacEwan, Gaius Cornelius, Gill09, Gogo Dodo, Habj, Hetar, Hu12, I dream of horses, Icairns, Isralegz, J.delanoy, JForget, JeffAMcGee, Jersyko, Jimwilsonline, Joepzander, John Foley, Jreither, Justice12, Jwri7474, Kai Barry 2, Karada, Kenlamance, Kentonmann, Kittybrewster, Kostisl, LawPratical001, Lawyers2arrogant, Lihaas, LilHelpa, Lioness298, Longhair, MAVaughn, Markruffolo, Matthew Stannard, Mhadj001, Michael H 34, Michael Hardy, Michaelfoti, Mintguy, Munrolaw, Mustafaa, Nightshadow28, Nwwaew, Occupational Illness, Ohnoitsjamie, Outlinesllc, PTiger1985, Parenttimenet, Paroxysm, Parramattacitylegal, Paul foord, Pepo13, Philip Trueman, Piotrus, Postdlf, PullUpYourSocks, Redgunners, Rich Farmbrough, Rj, Robert Dal, Ronels, Rsu, SAC, Sardanaphalus, Scribe 13, Searsmall, Simetrical, SiobhanHansa, Slp1, Smorgan30, Snumbers, Sole Soul, Solob, Spellcast, SteveofCaley, THF, Tajus12, TastyPoutine, The Nut, TheCustomOfLife, Times10, Titoxd, Whisky drinker, Wikidea, Wjohnsonva, Woer$, Workplaceadvocate, Yakoo, Yedhulaprakash, Yupik, Zodon, Zzuuzz, , 147 anonymous edits

Image Sources, Licenses and Contributors

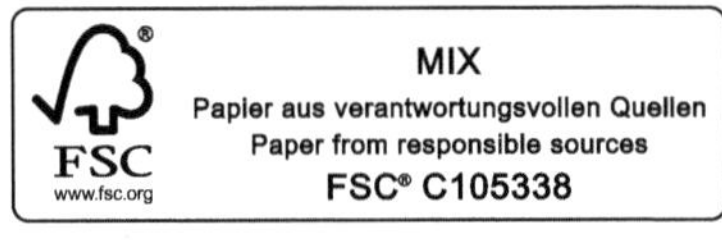